BRAIN MECHANISMS
AND BEHAVIOUR

The first edition of this book
appeared as

THE NEUROLOGICAL FOUNDATIONS
OF PSYCHIATRY

BRAIN MECHANISMS
AND BEHAVIOUR

An outline of the mechanisms of emotion,
memory, learning and the organization of
behaviour, with particular regard to the
limbic system

J.R.SMYTHIES

M.A. MSc. M.D. M.R.C.P. D.P.M.

Reader in Psychiatry, University of Edinburgh
Consultant Psychiatrist, Royal Edinburgh Hospital
and the Royal Infirmary, Edinburgh

CONSULTANT

W. ROSS ADEY M.D.

Professor of Anatomy
University of California, Los Angeles

SECOND EDITION

BLACKWELL SCIENTIFIC PUBLICATIONS
OXFORD AND EDINBURGH

SBN 632 06490 0

First Published 1966
Second Edition 1970

Printed in Great Britain by Alden & Mowbray Ltd
at the Alden Press, Oxford
and bound at Kemp Hall Bindery

CONTENTS

1 INTRODUCTION   1

   1.1 The current problem   1
   1.2 The development of concepts of higher brain functions   4
   1.3 Current research methods   6
   1.4 Some sources of complexity and error   7

2 NEUROANATOMY   13

   2.1 Some phylogenetic and developmental aspects   13
   2.2 Anatomical features of limbic structures   17

3 ABLATION AND STIMULATION STUDIES:
  THE EFFECT ON BEHAVIOUR   43

   3.1 The Klüver–Bucy syndrome   43
   3.2 The role of the amygdala   48
   3.3 The role of the hippocampus   63
   3.4 The role of the septum   75
   3.5 The role of the hypothalamus   80
   3.6 The role of the limbic midbrain area   86
   3.7 The role of various thalamic nuclei   88
   3.8 Miscellaneous regions   90
   3.9 The role of neocortex and juxtallocortex   93

4 SOME ASPECTS OF THE ELECTRICAL
  ACTIVITY OF LIMBIC AREAS   102

   4.1 The hippocampal theta rhythm   102
   4.2 The amygdala fast rhythm   109
   4.3 Feldman's hypothesis   111
   4.4 Seizure activity   112

5 THE LIMBIC SYSTEM, CONDITIONED
  REFLEXES AND LEARNING   113

   5.1 The various stages of conditioned reflex formation   113
   5.2 The role of different brain mechanisms in learning   123

v

6 MECHANISMS OF MEMORY   129

7 SOME NEUROCHEMICAL ASPECTS OF BRAIN
   FUNCTION   136

8 THEORIES OF FUNCTION OF THE LIMBIC
   SYSTEM   143
   8.1 Early theories   143
   8.2 The hippocampus   145
   8.3 The amygdala   152

9 SOME PSYCHIATRIC SPECULATIONS   158

   REFERENCES   170

   AUTHOR INDEX   180

   SUBJECT INDEX   184

Chapter 1

INTRODUCTION

1.1 The current problem

The present time is marked, in neurobiology and biological psychiatry, by rapid advances in our understanding of some of the brain mechanisms that underlie the control of emotion, of memory, of thinking and conditioned reflexes and of various aspects of motivation and behaviour. These aspects of things had traditionally been studied by psychological methods and their disorders in the field of clinical medicine have formed the bulk of clinical psychiatry. Thus the psychiatrist, in attempting to account for the origins and progress of the diseases seen in his clinic, has perforce to utilize explanations couched mainly in psychological terms, as in the current American fashion of psychodynamics, and the schools of thought based on learning theory; or in the mainly descriptive Kraepelinian tradition of British 'common-sense' psychiatry; or in sociological terms, as in some of the newer developments on both sides of the Atlantic. The bulk of psychiatry has remained descriptive. Schizophrenia, for example, is presented as a disease where emotional flattening, thought disorder, hallucinations and delusions simply occur together in different permutations and combinations. Manic-depressive illness consists of other contingent symptom complexes. The natural history of various types of neurosis are similarly described. However, in any developing science we must progress past the stage of mere description—the stage of natural history—and we feel that explanations must be given of why these illnesses develop in the people that they do and why they take the particular forms that they do: in other words we, as physicians, are expected to find out the aetiology of these illnesses. It has at any rate become clear that aetiology of psychiatric illness is usually multiple. Genetics, and developmental,

I

psychological and environmental factors play their part in nearly every case. Genetic factors determine the possible range of personality and liability to develop particular illnesses. If a person so predisposed happens to experience a faulty upbringing, for whatever reason and in various possible forms, and/or if in later life he is subjected to various forms of stress, these three factors acting in summation will determine if he develops a psychiatric illness and what form this will take. In individual cases the proportion of each factor will vary widely. In some cases of schizophrenia, for example, the genetic predisposition seems to be so strong that the illness develops in spite of an adequate upbringing and in the absence of a stressful life situation. In other cases of schizophrenia the operation of malign influences in childhood can clearly be seen to operate in the aetiology of the disease. Each individual factor can be regarded as contributing to the probability that the disease will develop, and the summation of these factors determines the course of events. Explanations of a psychiatric illness made in say psychodynamic or sociological terms in no way compete with, or contradict, explanations given in physiological or biochemical terms. They are complementary. Progress in our understanding in many of these fields is steadily being made; for example—biochemical factors in schizophrenia and other psychoses, the role of parental deprivation in childhood, the effects of social isolation, etc. But in the ultimate analysis what we do, the way we feel and how we think depends on the detail of events in the brain. Until very recently, however, hardly enough was known about how the brain engineers these functions to enable anyone to suggest what the physiological basis of any mental illness might be. The purpose of this book is to present what knowledge we have of these functions of the brain that may, by their disorder, be concerned in the aetiology of mental illness. Psychiatric symptoms are compounded mainly of disorders of emotion, memory, thinking and behaviour—in just those regions in which a great deal of work has been going on recently in neurophysiologial, neurochemical and psychophysiological laboratories. Yet this work is currently somewhat inaccessible for the clinical psychiatrist, or indeed for the neurobiologist who may be interested in finding out what is going on outside his own speciality. A number of excellent reviews have appeared (listed in 'References'), and I am indeed grateful to these reviewers who have assembled the truly vast literature in this field into a digestible form and on whose groundwork this book is based. But these are all limited in scope to one or other aspect of the field. There is no source where a general overall picture of these developments can be obtained such that a psychiatrist might like to have available. The difficulty here of course is the multitude of disciplines involved—neuroanatomy, neurophysiology, psychophysiology, neuropharmacology, psychopharmacology, neurochemistry, cybernetics, clinical neurology and psychiatry to name but the major ones. In view of the current vast expansion of these fields it becomes very difficult for any one person to gain an adequate working knowledge of developments in fields outside his own speciality. Yet each particular problem frequently has intricate and perplexing ramifications in many of these different fields. Several review volumes have appeared with different chapters written by specialists from these different fields. These are admirable for their own particular purpose but they are not suited for the present task which is to present a unified and comprehensive account for the non-specialist. Such a review needs to be written mainly by one person. It would seem desirable that psychiatrists should have a close understanding of our present knowledge of the cerebral basis of emotion, memory, mentation, motivation and behaviour.

The first edition of this book appeared under the title *The Neurological Foundations of Psychiatry* and the survey of literature for that was completed on December 31st, 1964. In the preface to that edition I suggested that a second edition would be necessary in two to three years' time in order to keep up with the rapid progress in this field. A sabbatical term spent with the Neurosciences Research Program of the Massachusetts Institute of Technology at the kind invitation of Professor Francis O. Schmitt provided the time necessary to bring the survey of the literature up to date. This was completed by the end of December, 1968 but the New York dock strike delayed the completion of the writing so that several later papers were able to be included. The review was carried out mainly in the most excellent library of the Harvard Medical School. The reader will notice the ever-increasing emphasis on chemical factors in the nervous system. In parallel to our developing understanding of the brain mechanisms at the level of the neurone, rapid advances are being made in the investigation into the molecular basis of synaptic function, of memory mechanisms and information processing in the brain. In order to avoid over-burdening the text with references and rendering it unreadable, a certain selection has been made. Well-established facts and research findings and theories have simply been presented: references have been reserved mainly for recent material or for material about which there has been lack of agreement.

I am grateful to the editors of the *Journal of Comparative Neurology* for permission to reproduce figures 6 to 11 and to Dr. Harold E. Himwich and Dr. Paul MacLean for permission to reproduce figures 12, 22 and 24.

1.2. The development of concepts of higher brain function

Not so long ago the general concept of the brain's function that most people accepted was based very much on Hughlings Jackson's doctrine of levels. The brain consisted, roughly, of a hind-brain, a midbrain and a forebrain. Primitive animals got along largely on the former. As evolution progressed more brain was added onto the front end of the nervous system to deal with the greater demands of the more complex environments of animals leaving the sea for land and of the pressure of natural selection. As each level of the nervous system developed it was supposed to take over the function, to a greater or lesser extent, of the more lowly ganglia, until, in man, all the higher functions were localized in the 'association' areas of the cortex. The thalamus seemed to exist mainly to shunt nervous impulses to the cortex and to subserve primitive forms of consciousness such as pain. The basal ganglia of the extra-pyramidal system seemed to be concerned mainly with refining and smoothing motor activity. The enormous complexities of what was then called the rhinencephalon were regarded as subserving the rather unimportant (for humans) sense of smell—forming as it were a vast cerebral veriform appendix. The hypothalamus was regarded as the main seat of the emotions subject to direct cortical control. The picture obtained of the main sensory inflow entering the various primary sensory areas. The messages were processed and passed to the surrounding cortex where they were 'elaborated' and were finally 'integrated', in the 'association' areas of the cortex that filled in the gaps between the specific sensory areas. Certain cerebral areas were recognized mainly on clinical grounds as dealing with specific higher functions; e.g. the frontal lobes with social factors, the parietal lobes with spatial functions, the temporal lobes with various complex sensory functions and emotion. The result of the complex interplay of schemata in the association cortices was finally fed by the transcortical fibre systems to the motor cortex—whereupon 'action' resulted—and to the hypothalamus—whereupon the appropriate emotions and their vegetative concomitants were evoked.

The major change that has taken place in the last twenty years or so has been the realization, based on evidence from a number of different sources, that the various ganglia lying at the base of the brain play an intrinsic part in higher mental functions of all kinds. The work of Moruzzi and Magoun showed how the activity of the reticular formation is essential for consciousness. This system produces widespread activation in the cortex and is responsible for behavioural and EEG arousal. 'In the minds of many neurophysiologists, the reticular formation has come to be regarded in much the same way as the cerebral hemispheres were envisaged in the nineteenth century' (Green, 1964). Then the work of Gastaut and his colleagues demonstrated the role of the intralaminar thalamic nuclei in the direction of attention. These interesting discoveries soon led people to take fresh note of the classical observations of Heinrich Klüver and Paul Bucy in 1937 on the syndrome named after them that results from bilateral removal of the temporal lobes in monkeys and in which changes in emotion, in memory and behaviour are prominent. People also recalled the theory put forward by James Papez at about the same time concerning the real function of one of the main features of the rhinencephalon—the great neural circuit provided by the hippocampus, fornix, mamillary bodies, mamillo-thalamic tract, anterior nucleus of the thalamus, cingulate gyrus and the cingulum that leads back to the hippocampus and so completes the circuit. Papez suggested that this circuit served not olfaction but the higher control of emotion.

It should be noted here that by 'circuit' one does not mean to convey an idea of a simply connected type of relay system. The system should allow for a series of complex transformations at each succeeding stage. There is, as yet, no clear evidence that a single stimulus can produce activity that can be traced through these successive pathways (Adey, 1965) but this may be because our stimuli are not physiological enough and our analysis of recordings too crude.

The extensive researches of Penfield and his school developed our understanding of the function of the temporal lobes, at least under certain specified conditions, as demonstrated by electrical stimulation in the conscious human subject.

These advances led physiologists and psychologists to turn their attention to the reticular formation (RF) and the limbic system (as the 'rhinencephalon' came to be called). In a very short time a vast literature appeared and it soon became apparent that the limbic system and related structures such as the hypothalamus, RF and the septal nuclei form a vastly complex and highly integrated system with further close connection with elements of the extrapyramidal motor system—particularly the caudate nucleus—various thalamic nuclei, and parts of the cortex; all closely concerned with aspects of 'higher' mental function.

1.3 Current research methods

1.3.1 NEUROANATOMY

New and refined methods of tracing fibre connections in the brain have been developed based on cutting the fibre tracts and tracing the subsequent degeneration of the distal axons to their termination. Most of this work has been done on animals and some details of these conclusions do not necessarily apply to man. However, general probabilities of human anatomy can be obtained by this method. In the human new techniques based on delineating fibre tracts by freezing have been developed and operations such as leucotomy give us occasional material that can be studied by degeneration methods. The emphasis in modern research has turned to histochemical methods of tracing specific chemically identified neurons and to electron microscopy, fluorescent and other microchemical methods, microautoradiography, etc.

1.3.2 NEUROPHYSIOLOGY AND PSYCHOPHYSIOLOGY

In this field of study the classical disciplines tend to overlap considerably. The traditional method of tracing functional connections by stimulating one nucleus or tract and finding out where the evoked potentials can be recorded from has been widely used. EEG methods have also been applied and the distribution, nature and the parameters governing the appearance of natural and evoked rhythms have been investigated together with such specific features as arousal patterns, seizure activity and so on. Ablation studies have determined the effect of removing parts of the brain on learning, emotion, conditioned reflexes and behaviour of all kinds. The development of techniques of putting indwelling electrodes into the brain and stimulation by radio has enabled psychophysiologists to study the effects of electrical stimulation of the brain on natural behaviour without the complicating effects of restraint, anaesthetics, etc. Likewise indwelling electrodes have enabled records to be taken of the electrical activity of the brain during many different kinds of behaviour. The use of the computer has extended the range of information that it is possible to extract from an experiment and thus has enabled more subtle experiments to be carried out. Again chemical methods of stimulation are coming into wider use.

1.4 Some sources of complexity and error

A great deal of information has been obtained by these methods and a clearer picture has emerged of how some of these brain mechanisms may operate and subserve these behavioural functions. However, there are naturally disagreements in the literature and some of the many difficulties inherent in this work should be mentioned before we go on to consider the information obtained.

1.4.1 SPECIES DIFFERENCES

There are often quite marked species differences in the quantitative and even qualitative function of various centres in the brain. For example the changes in delayed response performance following frontal ablations are prominent in monkeys, only temporary in chimpanzees and are not seen at all in humans (Rosvold and Mishkin, 1961). The hippocampal theta rhythm is a more complex phenomenon in cats than rabbits (Lesse, 1960; Adey, 1965). The details of the hippocampal and amygdaloid projections to septal and hypothalamic regions show differences in different species (Nauta, 1958).

1.4.2 ANATOMICAL DIFFERENCES

Then there are what we can call anatomical differences. Any lesion made at operation is likely to miss some of the target nucleus and may involve other unwanted nuclei either directly, or by damage to their blood supply, or to their fibre tracts that pass fortuitously through the nucleus concerned. Similarly in human cases of cerebral injury or tumour it is difficult to delineate the exact extent of the injury or tumour, or to judge the relative importance of associated oedema, hydrocephalus, propagated seizure patterns, etc.

The interpretation of ablation experiments is also difficult. Changes in function subsequent to the operation do not necessarily imply that the function is located in the part removed. The part may really function as an integral unit of a larger circuit of inextricably linked nuclei and tracts. The effects seen may be due to the release of lower centres from control, or to the irritation from scar tissue thus representing an exaggerated or distorted function of the part ablated rather than an absence of its influence. Gregory's (1961) simile will be recalled: if one removes a valve from a wireless set a melancholy wail may result. This does not indicate that the function of the valve was to suppress the melancholy wail. An example of conflicting claims based in part on differences of this kind are those made by some groups that lesions in the amygdala in cats makes them more docile whereas other groups report that this operation makes them more savage. Likewise experiments based on chemical manipulations are difficult to interpret—for example if we give a drug that inhibits serotonin mechanisms, a behavioural syndrome may result. But this may be due to the build-up of precursors of 5HT, or lack of its metabolites, or the unbalanced action of NE mechanisms, etc.

1.4.3 PHYSIOLOGICAL VARIABLES

'Physiological' variables that have been shown to be of importance in explaining why two groups doing what at first sight appears to be the same experiment get opposite results, have been such things as the anaesthetic used, the frequency and waveform of the electrical stimulation,* the age and previous training of the animal and the stage of learning reached, whether the stimulus excites the neural mechanism or 'jams' it, the propagation of the activity induced to other and interfering regions and so on. For example, Buchwald and Ervin (1957) claim that merely by altering the physical characteristics of the electrical stimulus used in stimulating one locus in the amygdala they were able to produce behavioural changes ascribed by previous workers as specific functions of different amygdaloid nuclei. Cortical evoked potentials in

---

* 'In describing effects of electrical stimulation one *must* indicate stimulus characters and parameters. Local brain stimulation in human frontal and limbic cortex rarely evokes any subjective sensation or change in behaviour unless one reaches the after discharge level when the effects become widespread. In the tiny animal brains the conditions are even more difficult unless one keeps to the threshold. The *volume* stimulated rises as the cube of the voltage' (Adey, 1965).

response to conditioned stimuli may get smaller or larger depending on how the animal was trained (Galambos, 1961). Stimulation of loci in the brain may either excite or inhibit other loci depending on the stage of learning reached (Morrell, 1961). Adey (1965) suggests '. . . any discussion of the effects of stimulation must necessarily consider the phenomena involved. It should deal with the inevitability of clamping a volume of tissue adjacent to the electrode itself, a surrounding area which is excited in a normal fashion, and beyond that a volume of tissues in the subliminal fringe. Each may be expected to establish its own gestalt through a series of widely located brain systems. In other words, I find singularly little in all the vast volume of stimulation studies of subcortical structures that would promote the notion of "centers". There seems to be the need to introduce the notion of complex cortical–subcortical interrelations, rather than the autonomy of activity in the sense of centers.'

Lastly, one must note that electrical stimulation necessarily involves a somewhat unphysiological means of evoking activity in the region concerned. We would be unable to discover much about the workings of a computer by passing large currents at random through its networks. But when we inject a chemical we know that it may diffuse extraordinarily rapidly especially if it is a physiological substance for which there may be specific uptake and conduction mechanisms.

1.4.4 PSYCHOLOGICAL VARIABLES

'Psychological' variables are even more complex. The apparent effect of lesions may depend on the situation in which these effects are looked for. For example a monkey with an amygdala lesion shows increased aggressiveness if tested in an individual cage situation but will change from a dominant to a submissive role if observed in a group hierarchy situation (Rosvold et al, 1954). Then again an animal stimulated say in the septal area may cease to respond to a conditioned stimulus, not because there has been any interference with the conditioning mechanism as such, but because the animal is 'enjoying' the pleasurable sensations evoked apparently by septal stimulation to the exclusion of attending to less interesting affairs outside. Likewise seemingly adverse reactions may be produced merely because we have stimulated low-level pain centres or pathways in the brain. There are also many factors in the behavioural situation that can exert an unsuspected effect as uncontrolled variables—e.g. the degree of energy that the animal must exert to achieve the response, whether the animal is under stress or not, its day-to-day handling by the laboratory staff, the degree of stimulus clarity, whether the stimuli were presented together or successively, etc. Then again a particular behavioural result may be produced by a different— usually more general—mechanism than that the experimenter may have supposed. For example, Weiskrantz (1956) points out that the observed effect of amygdalectomy on aggressive/defensive behaviour in monkeys where apparent tameness is produced, may not be due to any real effect on an 'aggression' centre but to a more general effect on the mechanism controlling conditioned reflex formation—in this case on rates of extinction. That is to say he supposes that the basic result of the amygdala lesion is to accelerate the rate of extinction of a previously learned conditioned fear response, without any change in the ability to acquire new conditioned learning. Thus, if the animal is handled kindly after the operation, the usual savage response of the monkey to man will be rapidly extinguished, whereas if additional adverse stimuli are introduced increased fear and aggression may be induced. The hypothesis is therefore that the amygdala does not control aggression as such primarily but it does control the rate of extinction of a conditioned avoidance response and that a secondary effect of the latter is a change in the aggressive permissive patterns of behaviour of the animal.

Another example is the current dispute over the 'real' function of the frontal lobe. Is this to enable the animal to delay a response so that it does not have to respond at once to the immediate stimulus? The test that illustrates this is the delayed response reaction. Here the animal is shown for example two cups under one of which a piece of food is placed. It is prevented from responding for some seconds. When allowed to the normal monkey can pick up the correct cup at once. The animal with both frontal lobes removed is unable to do so. Its delayed response has been affected. However, the frontal lesion could produce this result, not by affecting some delaying mechanism but by affecting sensory discrimination or memory; or by a failure to inhibit unwanted and competing responses. Or is the frontal lobe primarily concerned with primary drive inhibition? Or, as the clinical results of pre-frontal leucotomy suggest, with storage of certain social behaviour patterns? Or is it concerned with all of these in part, either on a regional basis or because of the functional relationship between these reactions—for example if an animal cannot delay its response to a stimulus it will be liable to be more distractible. Or do the results obtained depend largely on the accidental details of the training procedures used? And so on.

Chapter 2
NEUROANATOMY

2.1 Some phylogenetic and developmental aspects

Neuroanatomy, as it was taught until recently and as it still appears in many textbooks to this day, expended a great deal of energy and attention on the spinal cord, on the arrangements of tracts and nuclei in the brain stem and midbrain and on the thalamus, corpus striatum, cerebellum and cortex. Very little attention was paid to the hippocampus, amygdala and the rest of the 'rhinencephalon', presumably as they were regarded as the quasi-vestigial remnants of a system mediating the unimportant sense of smell. In the 1946 edition of Gray's *Anatomy*, the rhinencephalon is allotted four pages, much of which is taken up by figures. The amygdala and its connections rate half a page in the section on the corpus striatum.

In the developing brain the front end of the primitive neural tube forms the forebrain or telencephalon. The cells on the upper part of the lateral surface of this proliferate to form the two cerebral vesicles that expand rapidly on each side of the neural tube. The parts of this vesicle nearest to the hypothalamus, which is its medial surface forming a ring around the interventricular foramen, will form the future limbic system (see fig. 1).

The front end of the neural tube is provided by the lamina terminalis across the upper part of which grow the fibres of the anterior commissure just in front of the interventricular foramen. The choroid fissure and plexus that forms the roof of the IIIrd ventricle carries across the interventricular foramen to form the medial wall of the cerebral vesicle as this grows rapidly backwards. The olfactory bulb grows out of the anterior end of the inferior surface of the vesicle and the region immediately around its base becomes the future olfactory region of the cortex.

Just as the original neural tube developed local thickenings in its wall by neural migration and division to form the thalamus and hypothalamus, so the primitive cerebral vesicles develop thickenings on their lower halves to form the future corpus striatum in the lateral wall of the vesicle and the septal nuclei in an equivalent

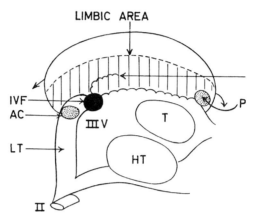

Figure 1. An early stage in the embryonic development of the forebrain

AC	Anterior commissure	LT	Lamina terminalis
CP	Choroid plexus	P	Pineal body
HT	Hypothalamus	T	Thalamus
IVF	Interventricular foramen		

position in the medial wall of the vesicle (fig. 2). Elliott Smith (1910) describes the situation in a hypothetical very primitive protomammal in the form shown in figure 2.

The developing neocortex displaces the hippocampal and amygdaloid formations to the medial aspect of the hemisphere as is shown in figure 3.

The continued development of the cortex pushes the posterior pole backwards and then downwards and forwards to form the temporal pole carrying part of the hippocampal formation and the archistriatum (amygdala) as well as the tail of the caudate nucleus with it (fig. 4).

The migration of the temporal pole from A to B in figure 4 inverts the relationship of the hippocampus to the archistriatum.

These, in the new position of the temporal pole, are now postero-ventral and anterodorsal respectively (see fig. 12). Thus the hippocampus in this part comes to lie on the inferior surface of the inferior horn of the lateral ventricle and the amygdala in the roof of the tip of the inferior horn.

In the human brain the enormous posterior growth of the corpus callosum from its origins just behind the hippocampal commissure carries the hippocampus on its dorsal surface (and

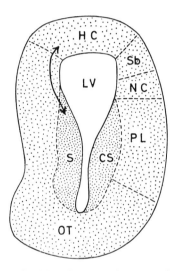

Figure 2. The cerebral hemisphere of a (hypothetical) prototype mammal (after Elliott Smith, 1910)

CS	Corpus striatum	OT	Olfactory tubercle
HC	Hippocampus	PL	Pyriform lobe
LV	Lateral ventricle	S	Septal nuclei
NC	Neocortex	Sb	Subiculum

reduces this pattern to the vestigial induseum griseum and longi-tudinal striae) and the fornix on its ventral surface. The septal nuclei remain in their original position in the medial surface of the hemispheres adjacent to the lamina terminalis and form the parolfactory area in man—the most posteromedial part of the frontal lobe cortex (and see section 2.2.1). The close direct original hippocampal–septal connections shown in figure 2 and the

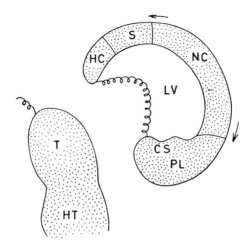

Figure 3.   An early stage in the embryonic development of the limbic system

CS	Corpus striatum	NC	Neocortex
HC	Hippocampus	PL	Pyriform lobe
HT	Hypothalamus	S	Subiculum
LV	Lateral ventricle	T	Thalamus

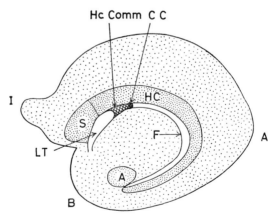

Figure 4.   The medial aspect of the brain of a primitive mammal (from H. E. Himwich)

A	Amygdala	HC Comm	Hippocampal commissure
CC	Corpus callosum	LT	Lamina terminalis
F	Fornix	S	Septum
HC	Hippocampus		

equally close hippocampal–hypothalamic and hippocampal–tegmental connections (that simply ran in front of the interventricular foramen), become converted into the long curved path of the fornix solely by this migration of the temporal pole. The amygdala gives evidence of its migration by the long curved path of the stria terminalis along the inner aspect of the caudate nucleus (fig. 12). The growth of the fibre tracts of the internal capsule cements the medial aspect of the cerebral vesicle to the lateral wall of the thalamus. This offers a second pathway for fibre tracts to connect the amygdala and hippocampus directly with the hypothalamus and reticular formation. Lastly the posterior part of the hippocampus rolls over on itself to give the familiar figure resembling a sea-horse.

The limbic system is present in all vertebrates and in most chordates. Amongst vertebrates only amphioxus is known to lack a well-developed limbic system. In phylogenesis there are animals with a brain stem alone, those with a brain stem plus a limbic system and those that add to these a neocortex. The limbic system is well developed in such animals as the whale and dolphin who lack olfactory nerves and man has the largest (relatively and absolutely) hippocampus of any animal.

2.2 Anatomical features of limbic structures

This brief outline of the development of these structures enables us to make some sense of their anatomical connections. On reading some of the current literature in neuroanatomy one sometimes gets the dismayed impression that everything in the brain is connected to everything else and that perhaps neuroanatomy should be written in terms of those structures that are *not* connected to each other! However this account will only take into consideration major pathways. The main structures that we shall be concerned with are (1) the hippocampus (HC) (2) the amygdala (3) the septum (4) the hypothalamus and preoptic area (5) certain thalamic nuclei (anterior, dorsomedial and intralaminar) (6) the midbrain tegmentum and reticular formation (7) various regions of the cerebral cortex (temporal lobe, orbito-frontal-insular cortex, cingulate gyrus, pyriform lobe) and (8) parts of the corpus striatum and subthalamus. Figure 5 gives a general picture of the limbic system. Adey (1965) emphasizes, however, that '. . . the most important connections in these cerebral systems are probably the multisynaptic paths that virtually defy any classical anatomical attempts to unravel them'. Mention of these diffuse multisynaptic paths will be made in due course, in particular those connecting amygdala and hippocampus with hypothalamus and brain stem.

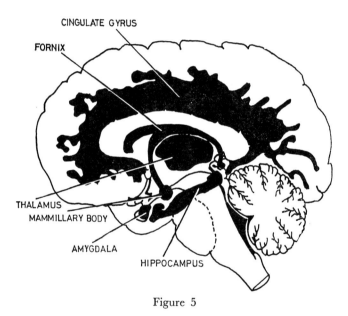

Figure 5

2.2.1 DESCRIPTION OF STRUCTURE

Some of these structures require a brief introductory description.

The hippocampus

This is merely the most medial portion of the cerebral cortex developed from the stalk, as it were, of the original cerebral vesicle. The dorsal half in man is reduced to a vestige by the growth of the corpus callosum but the ventral half abutting on the

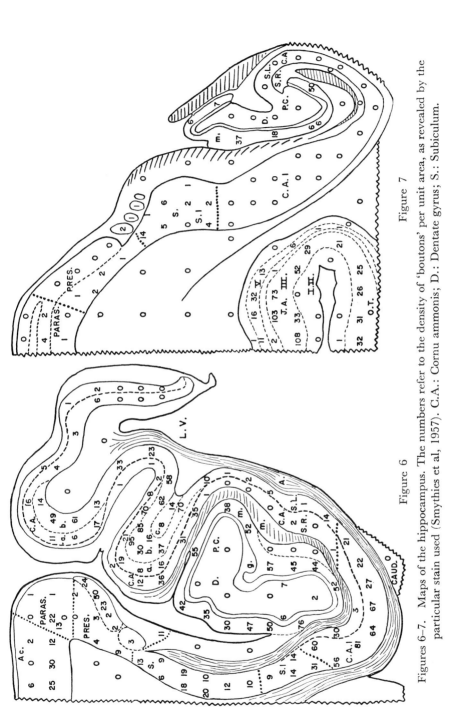

Figure 6

Figure 7

Figures 6-7. Maps of the hippocampus. The numbers refer to the density of 'boutons' per unit area, as revealed by the particular stain used (Smythies et al, 1957). C.A.: Cornu ammonis; D.: Dentate gyrus; S.: Subiculum.

inferior horn of the lateral ventricle remains. Its anterior portion—the pes hippocampi—remains an undulating piece of primitive cortex (allocortex) in the floor of the ventricle, whereas the posterior portion becomes rolled up on itself as the cornu ammonis in the form of the sea-horse. A portion becomes isolated from the rest to cap the cornu as the dentate gyrus. In neocortex the cells are arranged in six layers but in allocortex they form essentially one layer of large pyramidal cells. Their apical dendrites run parallel to each other into the superficial (or molecular layer) and their axons runs towards the ventricular surface where they form a layer of white matter—the alveus—that covers this surface. These axons then collect to form a bundle—the fimbria—that runs backwards along the edge of the hippocampus to form eventually the large bundle of the fornix. Some axons run the other way to distribute to the temporal lobe (see figs. 6 and 7).

The amygdala

This is a collection of nuclei situated at the anterior end of the roof of the inferior horn of the lateral ventricle in the white matter of the medial part of the temporal lobe. Anteriorly it is continuous with the cortex of the periamygdaloid area (an anterior division of the pyriform lobe and a part of the cortical olfactory area) and posteriorly it is continuous with the tail of the caudate nucleus. It is composed of a phylogenetically older portion—the medial and cortical nuclei—that have close olfactory connections, and a phylogenetically younger portion—the basal and lateral nuclei which are closely connected with the rest of the limbic system (figs. 8, 9 and 10).

The septum (or septal nuclei)

The main septal region in man is not the thin septum lucidum that fills in the gap between the corpus callosum and the fornix, but it is the subcallosal (parolfactory) area, a small region under the corpus callosum on the medial aspect of the frontal lobe (fig. 11). This area is the homologue of the medial septal nucleus of lower animals. The human homologue of the lateral septal nuclei is the thin plate of grey matter on the lateral surface of the septum pellucidum.

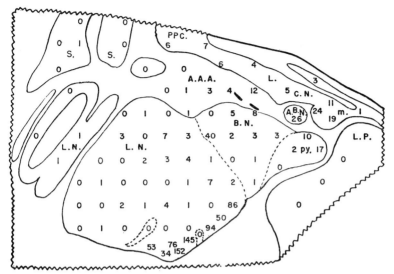

Figure 8

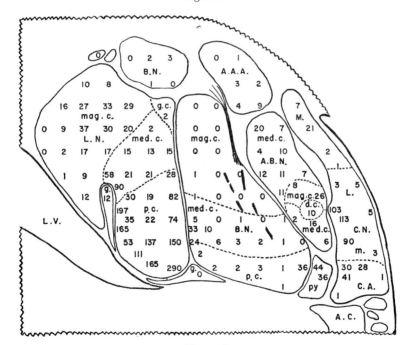

Figure 9

The septal area is thus merely the most medial portion of the frontal lobe (the paraterminal body) part of which retains its primitive position on the medial wall of the hemisphere and part of which is distorted by the growth of the corpus callosum and fornix. The septal area in man is continuous dorsally with the vestigial

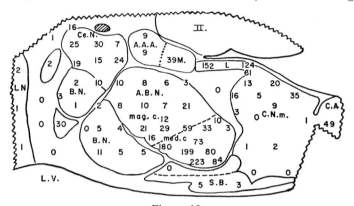

Figure 10

Figures 8–10. Maps of the amygdala
A.A.A., C.N., Ce.N., M.: portions of corticomedial group of nuclei
A.B.N., B.N., L.N.: portions of basolateral group of nuclei

dorsal hippocampus and medially around the interventricular foramen with the preoptic area and thence the hypothalamus, as one would expect from its developmental history.

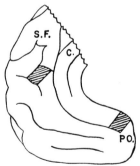

Figure 11. Map of medial surface of frontal lobe showing site of septal (PO) area in man
S.F.   Superior frontal gyrus   PO   Parolfactory (septal) area
            C.   Cingulate gyrus

The pyriform lobe

This is composed of the entorhinal area posteriorly and the periamygdaloid cortex and the prepyriform area anteriorly. It is merely the most medial part of the inferior surface of the temporal lobe comprising much of the hippocampal gyrus and adjoins the HC and subiculum (in its causal portion) and covers over the amygdala (and is continuous with the cortical nucleus of the amygdala) in its rostral portion.

The juxtallocortex

In between the allocortex of the hippocampus and subiculum and the neocortex of the temporal and frontal lobes there lies a zone of intermediate cortex—or juxtallocortex—with certain structural specificities. It includes the presubiculum, the cingulate cortex (also called 'mesocortex') and parts of the buried 'frontotemporal' cortex of the orbito-insular-temporal floor of the sylvian fissure.

The fornix

The fornix is a large bundle of fibres that originates from the HC (via the fimbria) and then sweeps upwards and then forwards following the course of the lateral ventricle (first on its floor, then posterior wall then roof) to dive into the septal area. Here it divides into two parts—the precommissural division that runs in front of the anterior commissure mainly to the septum; and the post-commissural division that runs posterior to the anterior commissure mainly to the preoptic area and hypothalamus. It carries fibres in both directions between HC, septum, hypothalamus and RF. Figure 12 gives a general picture of some of the main limbic structures and their connections.

The stria medullaris

This is a fibre bundle running a conspicuous course along the medial aspect of the thalamus just under the ependyma of the IIIrd ventricle. It joins an anterior group of nuclei (septum and fibres from the HC and amygdala) to the habenula which is an outlying thalamic nucleus close to the pineal gland. From here impulses are relayed to the dorsal tegmental region of the midbrain (closely linked to the RF).

The stria terminalis

This is mainly an efferent pathway from the amygdala. It emerges from the posterior end of this nucleus and follows the

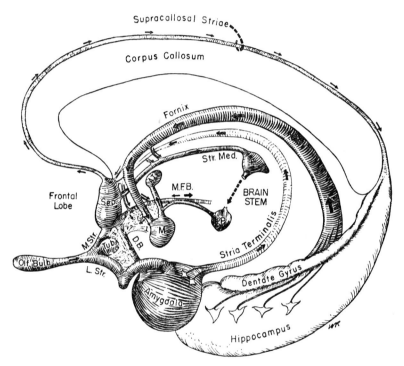

Figure 12.   A general picture of the limbic connections*
(from P. D. MacLean and H. E. Himwich)

* Code for abbreviations in figures 12–20 on page 42

tail of the caudate nucleus all the way round the lateral ventricle (first in the roof of the inferior horn and then in the floor of the lateral ventricle proper). It then enters the septal region. It carries fibres between the amygdala and the septum, hypothalamus and RF.

The medial forebrain bundle
The medial forebrain bundle (MFB) runs through the middle of the lateral hypothalamus and connects much the same nuclei as does the stria medullaris (including interconnections between many of the hypothalamic nuclei)—except that it by-passes the habenula and runs straight to the tegmentum to a region called the 'limbic midbrain region' (that includes the dorsal tegmental region) because so many limbic structures connect there.

The dorsal longitudinal fasciculus of Schulz
This connects the limbic midbrain area with medial hypothalamic nuclei and the intralaminar thalamic nuclei (thalamic portion of the RF).

2.2.2 THE CONNECTIONS OF THE LIMBIC SYSTEM*

The purely olfactory connections
The term 'rhinencephalon' originally connotated that this was the part of the brain concerned with olfaction. This once vast empire has now dwindled to a very small territory. The fibres from the olfactory bulb run via the lateral olfactory tract to the prepyriform and periamygdaloid cortices and to the cortical and medial nuclei of the amygdala, all situated close together on the medical surface of the anterior part of the temporal lobe (not far from the uncus). Impulses are conducted from here to the medial forebrain bundle and elsewhere. This comprises the extent that we know for certain of the primary olfactory cortical area. The primary olfactory cortex also receives fibres from the RF (including the intralaminar thalamic nuclei that probably subserve 'attention').

The connections of the hippocampus (fig. 13)
The HC has one very obvious fibre tract—the fornix. This was

---

* Section 2.2.2 is necessarily somewhat dry since there is no way to present anatomical connections except in this condensed form. The reader is invited to regard this section as an astringent aperitif for what is to follow.

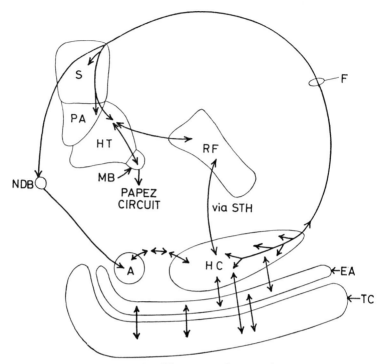

Figure 13.   Hippocampal connections

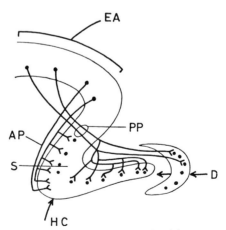

Figure 14.   The connections between the hippocampus and the
entorhinal area

AP	Alvear path	HC	Hippocampus
D	Dentate gyrus	PP	Perforant path
EA	Entorhinal area	S	Subiculum

at one time thought to be mainly efferent but it is now apparent that it has a strong afferent component to the HC as well. The main *afferent connections* to the HC are as follows:

(1) A pathway from the adjacent entorhinal area (hippocampal gyrus) that distributes via the alvear and perforant paths of Cajal to the dendrites of the pyramidal cells (fig. 14). This provides a pathway for impulses from the temporal lobe. There are extensive connections to the HC from all regions of the temporal neocortex. The behavioural function of this input is not clear for several reasons that will be discussed below (sections 4.1, 6.1).

There are two pathways from the entorhinal area to the CA 1 pyramids. The first is the direct monosynaptic pathway via the perforant path. The second has three synapses (dentate cell dendrites, CA 3 dendrites and Schaeffer collaterals). The wiring diagram of HC is shown in figure 15. In this the main input from the entorhinal cortex (perforant path) is shown

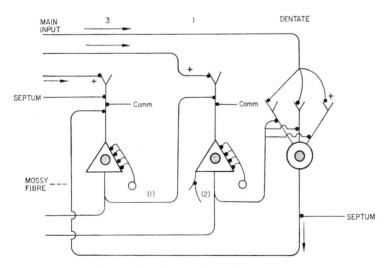

Figure 15. Wiring of the hippocampus

| 1 and 3 | Areas of cornu ammonis | (1) | Schaeffer collaterals |
| Comm | Commissural fibres | (2) | Commissural fibres and input from entorhinal cortex |

C

making synapses with the apical dendrites of the HC pyramids and dentate pyramids. The latter send their axons to the main dendrites of CA 3 pyramids (as mossy fibres). The alvear path from the entorhinal area runs to the basal dendrites of CA 1 pyramids. The axons of the HC pyramids form the efferent pathway and collaterals from the CA 3 pyramids run to the dendrites of the CA 1 pyramids. The input from the septum and the commissural fibres are as shown. The functional aspect of this diagram has been described by Gloor et al (1963). The main response to a volley of impulses in the afferent perforant path are EPSPs in the apical dendrites. These cannot fire the cells but serve to preset the trigger and allow the cells to be fired by the mossy fibres, whose apical dendrites are also stimulated by the perforant path volley. A delay circuit is provided by the Schaeffer collaterals. Lastly the basket cells (inhibitory interneurones) are activated to terminate all this activity. The input from the septum is strategically located to act as a gate for all this activity. Gergen and Maclean (1964) have suggested that this looks like a conditioning mechanism in which the fate of a volley in the afferent sensory performant path is determined by the visceral input from the septum. Clearly it could also operate on a matching device for comparing the input with selected items recalled from the memory store. The HC dendrites affect the soma by dendritic spike conduction rather than electronic spread (Anderson P. et al, 1966).

(2) The pathway from the RF running via the septum and fornix.

(3) Electrical studies in humans indicate the presence of a path from the thalamic RF.

(4) A two-way connection with the HC of the opposite side via the hippocampal commissure.

(5) A diffuse inflow from the limbic midbrain area via the subthalamic region. This may run via the septum in part.

(6) The cingulum from the cingulate gyrus and the medial frontal cortex.

The main *efferent connections* are:

(1) A major pathway that runs via the fornix to the septal region, the preoptic area, much of the hypothalamus, the limbic

zone of the midbrain RF, the dorsomedial and intralaminar thalamic (RF) nuclei and the mamillary bodies (and thence to the Papez circuit). Many of the fibres end in the septum and preoptic area and relay thence to the other structures in particular the dorsomedial and posterior hypothalamic nuclei. HC pyramids (intracellular recording) can be driven both orthodromically and antidromically by stimulation of the of the fornix (Green, 1964). The CA 1 pyramids in the anterior (dorsal) HC connect to the anterior thalamic nucleus and mamillary bodies and the CA 3 and CA 4 pyramids project to the septal region. The CA 1 cells of the posterior HC project to all these regions (Grant and Jarrard, 1968).

(2) An important pathway to the entorhinal area (Adey et al, 1956) (and thence by relay to the rest of the temporal lobe: Votaw, 1960). Lorente de Nò (1934) described how the axons of the hippocampal neurones bifurcate and send branches to the fornix route and to the entorhinal and temporal cortex.

(3) A direct route to the RF via the subthalamic area.

(4) There are diffuse two way connections with the ipsilateral amygdalae.

The septal path to the HC offers a means for activity ascending from the brain stem to reach the HC. In a conscious animal, as we shall see, an alerting stimulus induces a theta-wave response in the HC. This response is abolished by a septal lesion or by a lesion of the thalamic RF nuclei. Electrical stimulation of the septum easily gives HC responses. This path may not run along the fimbria on the surface of the HC (as the efferent HC fibres do) but may course in its depths to synapse on the granular cells of the dentate gyrus and thence relay to the HC pyramids. The dentate gyrus is in some respects the 'sensory' part of the HC and onto its individual granular cells converge afferent paths from many different sensory modalities including visceral afferents (Dunlop, 1958). HC pyramids can be driven by septal or entorhinal stimulation and by a variety of visual, auditory and tactile stimuli. Electrical studies show that the amygdala projects strongly to the HC, not directly, but via slowly conducting multisynaptic pathways running through the entorhinal cortex. Likewise HC seizures propagate readily to the amygdala (as well as to the RF and temporal neocortex). Functional relationships of the neocortex to HC have been investigated by Buresova et al (1962). They showed that putting the cortex out of action (by inducing spreading depression in it) caused changes in the rate of firing of single neurones in the HC (depression in 47·5 per cent, increase in 32·5 per cent). This increase was abolished by brain stem section suggesting mediation via the RF.

The HC takes part in several circuits which play a prominent part in the organization of the brain:

(1) The Papez circuit that we have described above.

(2) The circuit HC–septum–hypothalamus–RF. This can return to HC either by the same route or via the intralaminar thalamic nuclei or from RF to frontal cortex and then via the cingulum.

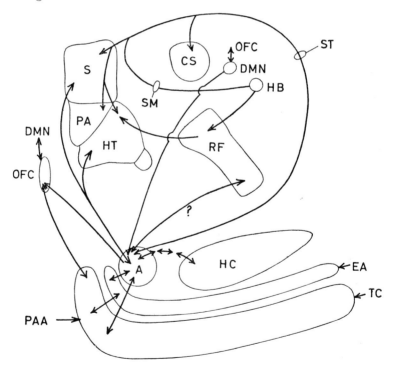

Figure 16.   The connections of the amygdala

(3) The circuit HC–entorhinal area–external capsule–anterior commissure–stria medullaris–RF–intralaminar thalamic nuclei–and back to HC. The first two would seem to be the most important ones.

The HC is a sheet of motor-like primitive cortex* interposed in a pathway mediating brisk streams of impulses passing in both directions between the temporal neocortex and juxtallocortex, the other important limbic structures (amygdala, septum and hypothalamus) and the RF (both in the midbrain and thalamus). Its possible functional role will be reviewed in the next section.

The dorsal and ventral HC have widely differing connections (Elul, 1964). The main afferents to both come from autonomic centres and the efferents return thither. There are also extensive connections with the entorhinal area and the septum. The dorsal HC projects mainly to cortical 'association' areas mainly in the temporal cortex and to the dorsal thalamic nuclei related to these.

The connections of the amygdala (fig. 16)

We have already dealt with the connections of the olfactory portion. The remainder, which is of interest to us in this connection, receives the following afferents:

(1) The surrounding temporal lobe neocortex and the cortex of the overlying pyriform lobe.

(2) A diffuse system from the anterior hypothalamus, preoptic and septal areas, and from the HC.

(3) The dorsomedial nucleus of the thalamus and (4) the RF via preoptic area connections.

Its *efferent supply* is widespread:

(1) Probably its most important efferents in man run medially, from the base-lateral group of nuclei as a diffuse projection to the anterior hypothalamus, preoptic region and septal areas. Fibres from the basolateral amygdala run mainly to the preoptic area and the paraventricular and ventromedial hypothalamic nuclei. The ventral pathway conducts many direct fibres from the pyriform cortex (as well as some from

---

* That is composed of large pyramidal cells in a relatively simple array.

here that relay in the amygdala) to the whole length of the medial forebrain bundle (MFB) region of the hypothalamus (Raisman, 1966).

(2) The stria terminalis carries fibres mainly from the corticomedial group of nuclei to the septal region, preoptic area and the mainly parasympathetic regions of the (anterior) hypothalamus (no fibres go to its ventral medial or dorsomedial nuclei. The impulses are then relayed by polysynaptic paths to the same 'limbic area' of the tegmental central grey (midbrain RF) as the HC projects to.

(3) Via the stria medullaris to the 'limbic area' of the midbrain RF with a relay en route in the habenula.

(4) To various thalamic nuclei (via the hypothalamus) including the dorsomedial nucleus and the intralaminar nucleus.

(5) Via the medial forebrain bundle to the lateral hypothalamus.

(6) To the caudate nucleus (particularly the nearest part i.e. the base of the head), the putamen and globus pallidus by direct pathways.

(7) To the amygdala of the opposite side via the anterior commissure.

(8) To the anterior half of the superior and middle temporal gyri, the ventral insular region and the caudal orbitofrontal cortex. There are connections between the inferior temporal gyrus and temporal pole with the cortical amygdala nucleus and the surrounding prepyriform cortex.

Thus the amygdala seems to have its main inflow from the temporal neocortex as well as from septal, hypothalamic and RF regions, and it has a very widely spaced outflow to the rest of the limbic system at various levels. There is much species variation in these connections.

The amygdala takes part in various circuits as does the HC. It has a very similar circuit running via septum, hypothalamus to RF and return as the corresponding HC circuit. Secondly the strong projection to the dorsomedial nucleus of the thalamus (present in monkey but not apparent in cat) gives a close connection between the amygdala and the orbitofrontal cortex. This in turn projects massively to the temporal neocortex and thence back to the amygdala. This recalls the HC circuit that runs to the anterior thalamic nucleus and thence to cingulate cortex (i.e. the Papez circuit). The dorsomedial nucleus also projects to the anterior hypothalamus and preoptic region and the orbitofrontal cortex projects via the medial forebrain bundle widely to subcortical structures (including the dorsomedial nucleus, hypothalamus and RF). There are thus widespread connections between the amygdala, dorsomedial nucleus of thalamus, and temporal and orbitofrontal cortex. There do not appear to be direct connections from orbitofrontal cortex to amygdala (in monkey) but there are probably connections via the preoptic region or temporal cortex.

The amygdala, like the HC, is sensitive to a wide variety of afferent inflow. There is much convergence from different modalities of sensation on to single units in the basal, lateral, central and anterior nuclei. The most effective stimuli are touch and sciatic nerve stimulation; then olfactory, then vagal and auditory stimuli and lastly visual stimuli. There was no such inflow on to any units in the cortical or medial nuclei demonstrating again the essential difference between these two nuclei and the rest of the amygdala. As in the case of the HC no particular part of the amygdala seems to be related to any particular part of the body.

Note the similarity between the afferent and efferent flows of the amygdala and the HC. Both lie astride connections between the temporal neocortex and subcortical limbic systems. Note again the similar circuits:

Thalamic nucleus	*Limbic cortex*
HC → anterior → cingulate → HC
Amygdala → dorsomedial → orbitofrontal → amygdala

Note also the other important circuits:

HC   → septal region → hypothalamus → RF → HC
  ⇅
Amygdala → septal region → hypothalamus → RF → amygdala

The connections of the septal area

This region of the brain, whose importance has only recently been given its true recognition, has marked two-way connections with the HC, amygdala, hypothalamus and RF just described. It will be recalled that the septum and the HC were once in close direct contact. Two rather specialized paths of the septal connections are the stria medullaris to the RF (via the medial nucleus of the habenula) and to the amygdala via the diagonal band of Broca. It also connects directly with the anterior, lateral reticular, dorsomedial and other thalamic nuclei, and cingulate gyrus.

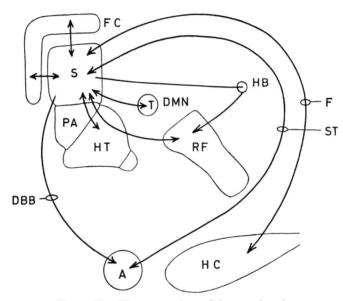

Figure 17.   The connections of the septal region

The connections of the hypothalamus and the preoptic area

We have already noted the important connections to the hypothalamus from the HC and septum (via fornix), amygdala (by two routes), the RF (by two routes) and the orbitofrontal cortex. The lateral area receives in addition fibres carried in the medial forebrain bundle from the caudate nucleus, substantia innominata and the pyriform lobe. The ventromedial nucleus receives the pallidohypothalamic tract from the globus pallidus. The main input and output of the hypothalamus involve the lateral area. The medial and ventral area communicate with the rest of the brain mainly via the lateral area (Bleier et al, 1966). Its efferent connections are:

(1) the medial forebrain bundle connecting with the orbito-frontal cortex rostrally and the RF and thence the visceral and motor nuclei of the brain stem and cord causally;

(2) The inferior thalamic peduncle connects to various thalamic nuclei and the mamillothalamic tract connects to the anterior nucleus;

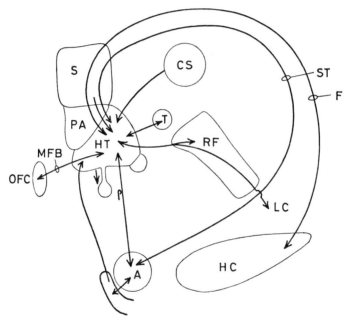

Figure 18. The connections of the hypothalamus

(3) The amygdala via the stria terminalis and a direct diffuse lateral outflow;

(4) the hippocampus via the septum and fornix;

(5) the habenula and RF via the stria medullaris;

(6) the infundibular region has important connections with the pituitary.

Stimulation in the septum and amygdala affects 60 per cent of neurones in the tuberal and lateral regions (Dreifuss and Murphy,

1968) and there is strong convergence between them. Seventy per cent of all neurones affected by septal stimulation were also affected by stimulation of the amygdala and these effects were synergistic in 83 per cent of cases. There was no difference in the direction of the effect between lateral and basal amygdala. Impulses from the HC and midbrain affected some 20 per cent of neurones in these areas and also converged on the 'septal-amygdala' neurones but not many were tested. The hypothalamus contains many different types of terminal, including dopamine, NE, 5HT as well as ACh ones. The dopamine terminals are very common in the dorsomedial nucleus and the medullary eminence. NE terminals are found particularly in the periventricular nucleus, the area between the ventromedial and lateral nuclei, the supra-optic and paraventricular nuclei and in the posterior hypothalamus. They are conspicuously absent from the mamillary nuclei and anterior area. 5HT is found in the suprachiasmatic nucleus.

The connections of the midbrain 'limbic region' (fig. 19)

As we have already seen the central grey matter of the midbrain has extensive limbic connections. This part is intimately associated with the RF and indeed is often merely called a part of the RF as a blanket name for the central grey matter of the midbrain and the tegmentum. Figure 19 shows a rough diagram of the anatomy involved.

The reticular formation (fig. 20) is very primitive phylogenetically and is initially derived from the grey matter around the central canal. It is composed of medullary, pontine, midbrain and thalamic regions. In the thalamus it comprises the intralaminar and midline nuclei (including the reticular nucleus). The main thalamic nuclei can be regarded as growing inside the RF and the latter is thus reduced in part to the parts dividing the main nuclei from each other (hence intralaminar). The septal region has been regarded as the rostral end of the RF. The RF is the central coordinating agent of the brain, as far as switching, modulating arousal, conditioning and general over-all control functions are concerned. It makes engineering good sense to have the central

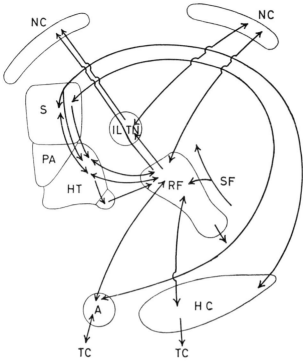

Figure 19.   The connections of the reticular formation

functional control system in so complex a mechanism as the brain in a central location.

The RF has many functions besides the limbic ones that we

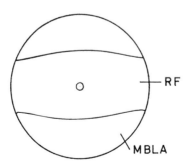

Figure 20 .   The relation of the limbic midbrain area to the reticular formation

shall be describing later. These include (1) its control of sleep and arousal (2) phasic and tonic motor control (3) modification of the reception, conduction and integration of all sensory impulses and (4) direct control of many visceral functions which shade off into its limbic function.

The 'limbic midbrain area' is divided into a dorsal and a ventral part. The ventral part consists of Tsai's ventral tegmental

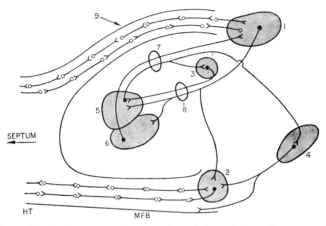

Figure 21. Main tegmental connections (adapted from Cowan et al, 1964)

1	Dorsal tegmental nucleus	7	Mamillotegmental tract
2	Ventral tegmental nucleus	8	Mamillary peduncle
3	Deep tegmental nucleus	9	Periventricular system
4	Tegmental reticular nucleus	MFB	Medial forebrain bundle
5	Medial mamillary nucleus	HT	Hypothalamus
6	Lateral mamillary nucleus		

area which is continuous anteriorly with the lateral hypothalamus, the interpeduncular nucleus, Bechterew's nucleus and the ventral tegmental nuclei of Gudden. These are all anterior to the red nucleus. The dorsal part consists of the ventral half of the central grey and the dorsal tegmental nucleus of Gudden. The main tegmental pathways are shown in figure 21.

This region receives a widespread afferent inflow:

(1) a massive projection from the hippocampus (via fornix as

well as a direct route of diffuse fibres running through the subthalamus;

(2) from the amygdala via the stria terminalis and intermediate relays in septum and hypothalamus;

(3) from the septum and hypothalamus via the stria medullaris, the medial forebrain bundle and the dorsal longitudinal fasciculus of Schutz;

(4) from the entorhinal area by a diffuse polysynaptic pathway running through the thalamus and hypothalamus;

(5) from various cortical regions including the cingulate gyrus, temporal neocortex and the orbitofrontal region—in fact the 'limbic areas';

(6) from the adjacent RF proper.

All these afferents overlap greatly with each other and with other RF afferents especially the diffuse (visceral) part of the spinothalamic tract, cerebellar and brainstem afferents. The only source of afferents to the dorsal tegmental nucleus is the mamillary body. Many fibres run to the ventral tegmental nucleus from the fornix and MFB. The main stream of classical sensory fibres, however, do not appear to be closely connected with the limbic midbrain area as they are, of course, with RF proper. (Note in this monograph RF stands for the RF proper and its more specific 'limbic' subdivision.) The main efferent limbic connections of the RF comprise:

(1) all the *hypothalamic nuclei* by two pathways (the ventral division to the mamillary bodies, lateral, preoptic as well as septal nuclei via the mamillary peduncle; and the dorsal division to the medial nuclei via the dorsal longitudinal fasciculus of Schutz);

(2) to the *hippocampus* directly (by diffuse connections running through the subthalamus) as well as by the septal-fornix route;

(3) to the *amygdala* by the septal route and the *entorhinal area* via the stria terminalis;

(4) to the *intralaminar thalamic nuclei* and of course widely to *cerebral cortex*.

Many RF cells have an axon that divides into a long branch running rostrally towards the direction of the thalamus and a caudally directed branch running towards the cord. Each cell has a very large number of synapses and there is extensive sensory, cortical and limbic (and other) convergence on each cell.

Stimulation of the interpeduncular nucleus in the rat leads to an 'obstinate' progression syndrome (Thompson and Rich, 1961) and the nucleus may be a non-specific relay centre for correlating visceral and sensory information (Plante, 1969).

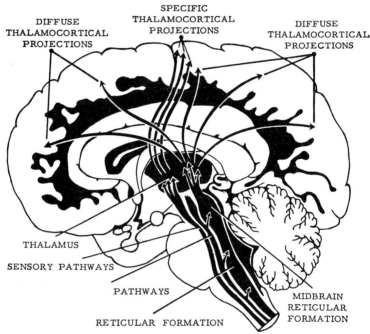

Figure 22.   The connections of the reticular formation and neocortex
(from H. E. Himwich)

Certain thalamic nuclei

The *non-specific group* (midline and intralaminar). These form a part of the RF and are concerned amongst other things with the function of selective attention. They receive an afferent inflow from the midbrain RF, the HC, amygdala, septum, all the cortex and by collaterals from the classical sensory pathways and from other thalamic nuclei. Their efferent outflow goes to the cerebral cortex including all the limbic cortex, all other thalamic nuclei, the HC and basal ganglia. This outflow is probably polysynaptic and goes via N. ventralis anterior and the reticular nucleus. The outflow to the cortex goes mainly to the superficial layers to axo-dendritic synapses.

The habernular nucleus. This receives the termination of the stria medullaris and it projects in turn by a compact bundle to the interpeduncular nucleus (and thence to the limbic midbrain area) and by a diffuse system to the midline thalamic nuclei and the central and lateral regions of the midbrain. The limbic connections of the other two 'limbic' thalamic nuclei—the anterior and the dorsomedial—will be clear from the account already given.

The limbic areas of the neocortex

The *temporal neocortex* (besides its specific auditory connections) connects with the following (fig. 22):

(1) the HC and amygdala (and thence to septum, hypothalamus and RF). The possibility of diffuse multisynaptic connections between these loci—with equivalent functional importance to the more obvious anatomical circuits described—should not be overlooked.

(2) The following thalamic nuclei—N. lateralis posterior, the pulvinar and the intralaminar group.

(3) Much of the extrapyramidal system.

(4) The midbrain tegmentum.

(5) The frontal lobe via the uncinate fasciculus.

The *cingulate cortex* consists of an anterior granular (motor-type) part and a posterior granular (sensory-type) part. It receives afferents from the anterior nucleus of the thalamus and from limbic and immediately adjacent neocortical areas. It projects to the anterior and other thalamic nuclei; to the HC via the cingulum; to the hypothalamus; to the caudate nucleus and globus pallidus to adjacent neocortical areas and for a diffuse path to brain stem (Ward, 1948).

The *orbitofrontal cortex* connects mainly with the dorsomedial nucleus of the thalamus, and with the hypothalamus and RF via the medial forebrain bundle which starts in this region and runs

back to the RF. The medial frontal cortex projects powerfully via
the cingulum to the HC.

Abbreviation for figures 12–20

A	Amygdala	MFB	Medial forebrain bundle
AT	Anterior nucleus of	NC	Neocortex
	thalamus	NDB	Nucleus of the diagonal
CS	Corpus striatum		band
DMN	Dorsomedial nucleus	OFC	Orbitofrontal cortex
EA	Entorhinal area	P	Pituitary
DBB	Diagonal band of	PA	Preoptic area
	Broca	PAA	Periamygdaloid area
F	Fornix	RF	Reticular formation
FC	Frontal lobe neocortex	S	Septum
HB	Habenular nucleus	SM	Stria medullaria
HC	Hippocampus	ST	Stria terminalis
HT	Hypothalamus	STH	Subthalamus
IP	Interpeduncular nucleus	T	Thalamus
MB	Mamillary bodies	TC	Temporal lobe neocortex

Chapter 3

ABLATION AND STIMULATION

STUDIES

3.1 The Klüver–Bucy syndrome

One (apparently) simple method of finding out what a part of the brain does is to remove it, or damage it and see what happens. This method has in fact many complications and difficulties that have been outlined in Chapter 1, but it has been extensively used in this field of enquiry. The effects of such damage can be determined in various ways such as the electrical activity of other parts of the brain, on some other physiological variable or on behaviour.

The classical research in this field was carried out by Heinrich Klüver and Paul Bucy (Klüver and Bucy, 1936, 1938, 1939). They removed both temporal lobes including HC and amygdala from monkeys and observed the behavioural effects. They noticed the following results that make up the Klüver–Bucy syndrome:

(1) *'Psychic blindness'*: the animals appeared to lose their appreciation of the meaning of objects and they would pick up without fear life-like models of snakes, which no normal monkey would ever do, or they might try to eat inappropriate objects such as pieces of iron.

(2) *Tameness*: the normally very aggressive monkeys became quite tame and easy to handle.

(3) *Hypersexuality*: the monkeys showed more sexual behaviour of various kinds.

(4) *Oral tendencies*: they showed an excessive tendency to put anything moveable into their mouths.

(5) *Hypermetamorphopsia* which is the tendency to shift their attention from object to object in a mechanical stereotyped manner.

It should be noted that many of the features of the Klüver–Bucy syndrome were described in 1888 by Brown and Schaeffer. They removed both temporal lobes in one monkey and noted the tameness, the loss of recent memory and the 'psychic blindness'. They obtained the same result in the case of another monkey in which only the superior temporal gyri were removed. However, the authors felt that there had been extensive vascular damage at operation to the rest of the temporal lobe and adjacent brain. In fact this consideration led them to fail to recognize the specific nature of their findings with respect to the temporal lobe, and they attributed their results to 'idiocy' induced by general cortical damage. It is remarkable that fifty years were to elapse before anyone recognized the true significance of their results.

Since the war a good deal of research has been directed towards a further analysis of this syndrome both in terms of a refined behavioural analysis—i.e. what deficits do these animals really show—and towards a better understanding of what role the various brain structures removed in a temporal lobectomy play (see the review by Adey, 1959). The present situation is as follows. The changes in perception seem to be a compound of two factors; (1) subtle disorders of visual discrimination due to removal of sensory analysers in the ventral temporal neocortex and (2) disorders of recent memory due to removal of the HC. Removal of these temporal gyri leads to various disorders of visual discrimination and removal of the pyriform lobe, amygdala and hippocampus leads to the production of the elements of the Klüver-Bucy syndrome without the gross sensory deficits. However, the functional relation between cortical structures and their connected subcortical structures is always close and complex and their function *is usually closely* dependent on each other, and indeed they may be thought to function as one unit. Thus it is easy to understand why bilateral removal of all the temporal neocortex (sparing the primary auditory cortex) with minimal damage to subcortical structures or entorhinal cortex produces many of the elements of the Klüver–Bucy syndrome—i.e. the expected sensory deficits, but also increased tameness, oral tendencies and a loss of fear of dangerous objects (Akert et al, 1961). These authors note the extensive connections between the temporal neocortex and the limbic structures and they postulate two varieties of the Klüver–Bucy syndrome (*a*) neocortical, which is transient and (*b*) limbic which is more permanent.

Stepien et al (1960) suggest that the 'oral tendencies' in these animals is really due to loss of recent memory. 'The animal (monkey) investigates these objects as a normal monkey would, but keeps on doing so as if unable to record previous experience. This lack of recent memory could also be shown by offering the animal a lighted cigarette which it would repeatedly take into its hands and burn itself.' They reported no true psychic blindness nor hypersexuality in their animals. The monkeys became somewhat tamer but showed rage reactions under certain circumstances e.g. when touched. They also ate abnormal foods such as meat.

Hypersexuality has resulted from lesions of the posterior part of the pyriform lobe alone (Green et al, 1958a, b). Removal of the HC and amygdala alone does not induce this effect. It has also been shown to respond to endocrine factors since it is abolished by castration and can be reintroduced by testosterone injections (Schreiner and Kling, 1954). The effect was not constant as it occurred in only 20 out of 82 operated cats. It was seen only in males who showed both excess normal sexual activity and abnormal forms of sexual behaviour, e.g. attempting to copulate with any furry object and exhibiting sexual behaviour outside their normal territory. These latter changes were not due simply to higher blood levels of testosterone since administering testosterone to normal cats did not result in this abnormal behaviour. A normal level of blood testosterone was, however, necessary for the aberrant behaviour to occur. Green et al (1958a) suggested that a disorder of perceptual mechanisms might be responsible for these results and that this part of the pyriform lobe in cats acts as a mechanism for correlating sexual behaviour with environmental stimuli as well as a more general function of inhibiting certain hypothalamic mechanisms. Some of the other facets of the Klüver–Bucy syndrome have also, it will be recalled, been attributed to disorders of perceptual mechanisms or of mechanisms concerned in the selection of appropriate behaviour to a given set of stimuli.

Lesions in the anterior portion of the pyriform lobe lead to hyperphagia but not to hypersexuality (Green et al, 1958a, b).

The problem of the control of aggressive behaviour is complex, and concerns particularly the amygdala, hypothalamus and RF. Most reports claim that damage to the amygdala causes a decrease in aggression and generally tamer behaviour. However some investigators have reported the opposite. Bard and Mountcastle (1948) removed the amygdala and the overlying pyriform lobe and produced very savage animals. The importance of cortical-limbic relations was shown by the fact that removing all neocortex sparing limbic structures induced 'placidity' and in these animals removing the amygdala and/or the cingulate gyrus restored aggression. Removal of the cingulate gyrus in normal cats however raised the rage threshold. Bilateral removal of the hippocampus and presubiculum in normal cats produced little change in this respect.

How can we explain the fact that some investigators report increased aggressiveness after amygdalectomy and some decreased? It is possible that the reason may be merely anatomical—i.e. that parts of the amygdala may potentiate aggression and other parts may inhibit it and that the different investigators have merely damaged different parts. For example Wood (1958) claimed that lesions limited to the basal nuclei of the amygdala led to increased aggression. The problem of functional differentiation within the amygdala will be considered further below (section 3.2). Kling et al (1960) carried out bilateral removal of the amygdala and pyriform cortex in cats. Most became tamer but two became very savage and one 'fearful'. These results did not depend on the previous 'personality' of the cats. It is also possible that the social conditions under which the experiments were done made a difference. Rosvold et al (1954) noted that their monkeys after operation were more aggressive if observed in their home cages but when they were in the presence of other monkeys previously dominant animals became submissive. Similarly dogs with pyriform–amygdala–HC lesions (Fuller et al, 1957) were less responsive than normal to stimuli and less timid in response to human beings but in a competitive feeding situation they were, the experimenters considered, merely indifferent which might have been misinterpreted as being 'timid'. Green (1958a) described amygdalectomized cats as 'fearful' rather than 'aggressive'. Bard in this same discussion disagreed. Green et al (1958a) point out that rage and fear reactions can be readily confused, as can indifference, catatonia, stupor, and idiocy. Thus the need for a more exact analysis of the behaviour manifested under controlled conditions becomes clear. The quantitative ethological techniques of Chance and Silverman (1964) would seem to offer advantages here. Another explanation is given by Schreiner and Kling (1954) who observed post-operative savage behaviour in cats only following an initial period of docility. This appeared to coincide with the onset of hypersexual behaviour. They suggested that the return of aggressive behaviour might be consequent upon the hypersexuality for these two aspects of behaviour are closely linked in carnivores: both were abolished by castration. Against this it must be noted that the cats of Spiegel et al (1940) were savage immediately after the operation and Bard and Mountcastle (1948) never observed hypersexuality in their (very savage) cats. In other series the aggressive behaviour started some time before the hypersexual behaviour. Furthermore, operations on the limbic system can be followed by a transient period of apathetic behaviour. Green et al (1958a) also linked the aggression with frustrated sex drive. Possibly the two are related in some but not all cases: that is hypersexuality can be a sufficient condition for the manifestation of aggressive behaviour but it is not a necessary one.

However, the appearance of the Klüver–Bucy syndrome does not appear to be entirely constant. Orbach et al (1960) did extensive removals of the amygdala, HC and HC gyrus in seven monkeys. The elements of the syndrome were only seen transiently if at all. Only one monkey showed hypersexuality. Excess orality occurred in all but transiently: in only one was it chronic. These differences presumably derive from the many variables inherent in these investigations that we have discussed. Another difficulty in interpreting these results has been raised by Green (1958b) in that lesions of the amygdala tend to lead to vascular damage involving nearby regions.

Lastly Weiskrantz (1956) has suggested that the amygdala does not control 'aggression' or 'placidity' as such but that it does so indirectly by controlling the basic mechanisms of conditioned reflex formation and in particular with reinforcement and extinction. This means that an amygdalectomized animal becomes tamer because his conditioned fear reaction to humans has undergone a much more rapid rate of extinction than usual. This suggestion will be considered in more detail below (section 3.2.3).

Other regions involved in the aggressive reactions are the hypothalamus and the RF. Lesion of the ventromedial nucleus of the hypothalamus results in extremely savage animals and this results even in the case of a placid animal with a previous amygdala lesion. This effect is presumably due to the unbalanced activity of the rage-producing hypothalamic centres. In other cases amygdala lesions can abolish this savage behaviour presumably acting via the hypothalamus.

The Klüver–Bucy syndrome has been induced in man by removing both temporal lobes (Terzian and Ore, 1955). It is similar to the syndrome seen in the monkey but shows the following differences: (1) there are no oral tendencies. This is presumably due to the fact that monkeys normally use their mouths to explore new objects and humans do not. In fact as we have seen it is probably a mistake to call this 'increased oral tendencies' when the real defect seems to be a loss of immediate memory. (2) An extensive loss of recent memory is very evident as well as impaired language function and alexia. There may be a complete loss of recognition of people, even of close relatives. Interest is limited to immediate needs and there is poverty of expression and loss of all emotion and aggressive behaviour. (3) There is no 'psychic blindness' (visual agnosia). Again this is probably a result in monkeys of loss of recent memory.

3.2 The role of the amygdala

We can now proceed to deal in more detail with the possible functions of individual elements of the limbic system as revealed by ablation and stimulation studies. We have already seen that the amygdala is concerned in some way with the control of aggressive responses, the pyriform cortex with sexual responses, and so on. It is known that decerebrate animals with hypothalamus and midbrain intact are capable of crude emotional responses. A midbrain animal will show rage reactions and will struggle to escape from painful stimuli. These regions are capable of organizing undifferentiated patterns of emotional behaviour lacking direction or relevance to the (external) situation. For example, the rage elicited is not directed toward any object, the struggle to escape pain is unaccompanied by any more complex activity to avoid the situations liable to lead to pain; the emotional expression is unconnected with the external situation. The extensive limbic connections with neocortex, hypothalamus and central midbrain regions (RF) suggest that this system mediates higher control of the hypothalamus and of emotional and autonomic responses and in particular the relevance of the behavioural and emotional responses to the environment in all its complexity of meaning and significance for the organism and its needs.

3.2.1 STIMULATION STUDIES

Electrical stimulation of the amygdala in animals gives rise to a variety of responses.

Somatomotor reactions

Stimulation of the lateral division (mainly) gives movements of the eyes, head, face and jaw. These may be tonic or clonic. There may also be arrest of spontaneous movement.

Visceral reactions

These (mainly from the medial division) include cardiovascular reactions of various kinds, respiratory inhibition, salivation, lacrimation, sneezing, changes in gastric acidity and motility, urination, defaecation, piloerection, pupillary dilation, erection, ovulation, uterine changes, premature labour and behavioural arousal. Some of these appear to represent isolated fragments of feeding, emotional and sexual behaviour. Stimulation of the amygdala can affect the amount of food intake, temperature regulation and sleep–activity cycles.

Behavioural reactions

The main behavioural effect obtained by stimulating the baso-lateral division of the amygdala in the intact unanaesthetized animal is the 'searching response'. This commences with the immediate arrest of all on-going activity. The animal raises its head, the eyes open wider, pupils dilate, ears erect, and its whole attitude becomes one of expectant attention. It then gives orienting movements which consist of quick searching movements of eyes, head and neck usually directed toward the opposite side. More intense stimulation gives rise to fear or aggressive/defensive reactions (Ursin and Kaada, 1960a, b). Bagshaw and Benzies (1968) showed that there are two separable components of the orienting response. Lesions of the amygdala abolished the GSR, heart rate, respiration rate and EEG changes but had no effect on the ear movement and the other motor components. In cats stimulation of the basolateral nuclei has been reported to induce cowering or attentive responses whereas stimulation of the central and medial divisions gave rage responses with increased gastric secretion and motility, and, in hormonally primed animals, ovulation, sexual excitement and uterine contractions. Stimulation of the lateral division has been reported to depress the rage reaction induced by hypothalamic stimulation. Thus it would appear that the medial amygdala was more concerned with eliciting rage reactions and the lateral division with inhibiting them. This role of the amygdala has been clarified to some extent by Egger and Flynn (1963). They used rather placid laboratory cats who would normally ignore a live mouse placed in their cage. Under these circumstances electrical stimulation of the lateral hypothalamus led to an immediate, well-directed and effective attack on the mouse. However, simultaneous stimulation of the basal nucleus and of the medial part of the lateral nucleus of the amygdala suppressed this hypothalamically elicited attack whereas stimulation of the dorsolateral part of the latreal nucleus facilitated it. The former effect was the more marked. Ursin and Kaada (1960a, b) also argue for some functional localization within the amygdala. The searching response in their series (cat) could be elicited from the basolateral division (as well as from various thalamic nuclei—intralaminar, dorsomedial, anterior—i.e. the 'limbic' ones) and fear and anger from the same sites at higher voltage. Autonomic responses resulted mainly from stimulation of the anteromedial group of nuclei.

The concept of the amygdala as composed of two carefully balanced and mutually antagonistic systems is supported by some neuropharmacological studies of Grossman (1964 a, b). In rats deprived of food and water direct adrenergic stimulation of the ventral amygdala leads to an increase of food and to a decrease of water intake. An adrenergic blocking agent had the reverse effect. There was no response in satiated rats. In the hypothalamus the effect of such stimulation was the same in both satiated and deprived rats. This suggests again that the amygdala is concerned with the higher control of the hypothalamus and with the reinforcing value of stimuli under different conditions of the environment (in this case of the internal environment). Other workers (Fernandez de Molina and Hunsperger, 1962; Hilton and Zbrozyna, 1963) confirm that stimulation of the amygdala leads to the defence reaction. This has an autonomic component (pupillary dilation, pilo-erection and muscle vasodilation) and a behavioural component manifest at greater stimulus strength (growling, hissing, ear retraction, claw extension, progressing to 'running wildly around the observation cage, jumping up the walls and urination if the bladder was full'). However no report is given of the reaction to humans, other cats, mice, etc.

The former workers claim that the efferent path for this reaction is the direct amygdala–hypothalamic pathway and that the only role of the stria terminalis in this is afferent to the amygdala. The brain stem also seems to be involved as unilateral coagulation here abolished the growling and hissing response obtained by stimulation of the ipsilateral amygdala but there was no effect on this reponse obtained by stimulating the contralateral amygdala. Bilateral coagulation of this zone of the midbrain produced its usual effect—an extremely unresponsive and inactive animal.

A note of caution has been sounded however by Buchwald and Ervin (1957) who claim to have evoked, merely by varying the parameters of the electrical stimulus used in a single site in the basolateral amygdala, the whole gamut of behavioural responses reported by other workers to be functions of specific subdivisions of the amygdala. However, here factors of differential current spread may be involved. Likewise Murphy et al (1967) state '. . . a division of the amygdala into functional compartments based on behavioural, endocrine or autonomic responses resulting only from high frequency stimulation of the amygdala may be premature.' They stress the marked differences in the effects obtained by varying the frequency and strength of the stimulus.

Thus the rage–aggression–defensive response may not depend on one 'centre' but on a system of connected loci in the amygdala, hypothalamus and RF. Within this there may be possible hierarchical or complementary 'push–pull' relationships as well as functional regional specialization but the number of uncontrolled variables in the work reported so far do not enable us to say much more than that.

In female rats electrical stimulation of the corticomedial amygdala leads to delayed puberty (Bar-Sela and Critchelow, 1966). The central and medial nuclei are positive reward centres in Olds's sense.

3.2.2. ABLATION STUDIES

The various somatomotor and autonomic mechanisms so clearly influenced by amygdala stimulation only show minor and transient, if any, disturbances following bilateral destruction of the amygdala. However, marked emotional and behavioural changes can be observed as was described in the section on the Klüver–Bucy syndrome. It should also be noted that different results from operations on the amygdala (and indeed on other structures) may be noted at different times after the operation. For example, for the first few days a sleep-like, or cataleptic-like, state is common. Then aggressive behaviour may develop after some days and sexual changes after some weeks. These changes tend to clear up in the reverse order. The effects of lesions in the amygdala can vary much according to the age of the animal and the species. In adult rats, for example, the main effects are aphagia and adipsia leading to death in two weeks if not fed. Males show no sexual behaviour but females are not affected although none managed to raise their litters. In infant rats the operation leaves no permanent effects. In agouti there is marked taming and no effect on the food intake. Wild cats are tamed; tame cats do not show this effect, but they show an increase in sexual behaviour, as do monkeys. In kittens and infant monkeys again there is little effect (Kling, 1966). Bilateral lesions in rats depress emotional reactions and increase exploratory behaviour (Allikinets and Lapin, 1967).

3.2.3 THE AMYGDALA AND LEARNING

The amygdala also appears to play a role in learning and in conditioning. Owing to the large number of potentially uncontrolled variables in learning and conditioning experiments there is plenty of scope for apparently conflicting results. Some workers have reported that amygdalectomy impairs the ability to *acquire* a conditioned avoidance response (CAR) (e.g. Robinson, 1963; Horvath, 1963; Weiskrantz, 1958): others that it does not (King, 1958; Weiskrantz, 1956). Some report that it affects the *retention* of a previously learned CAR (e.g. Pribram and Weiskrantz, 1955; Horvath, 1963; Ikeda, 1961): others that it does not (Weiskrantz, 1958). A more subtle approach is indicated by Weiskrantz (1956) who observed that amygdalectomy produced no very marked effect on a previously acquired CAR nor on the ability to acquire a new CAR but it did produce a very rapid rate of *extinction* of a previously learned CAR.

Horvath (1963) found the cats with bilateral amygdala lesions had impaired acquisition and retention of a CAR. He tested them both for an active CAR (where an animal must learn to escape from a particular locus on receiving the conditioned stimulus (CS)) and for a passive CAR (where the animal must learn to avoid going to a certain locus, e.g. to its food box which is intermittently electrified and the CS is a signal that the current is on). There was a good deal of individual variation amongst animals, and cats that were bad at learning the former might be good at learning the latter. Therefore he supposed that his results could not be due merely to a decrease in fear motivation. Horvath then put forward the hypothesis that the basolateral division of the amygdala might be part of a motor-facilitatory system (rather like the corpus striatum or cingulate gyrus) whose loss might impair active motor behaviour but not the mere inhibition of behaviour (some further evidence on this point is contained in the next section). However, the passive avoidance test was much *easier* than the active test and when Horvath used an easier active CAR amygdalectomy no longer had any effect. So he suggested the amygdala might be concerned with the acquisition of avoidance responses appropriate to situations of a higher order of *complexity*. Lesions of the rostral part of the lateral amygdala depress active avoidance learning, and lesions of the medial part depress passive avoidance learning. Ursin (1965) points out that these two types of avoidance response depend on two different innate response patterns reciprocally related and modulated by the amygdala: (i) fear leading to flight and (ii) fear leading to a freezing reaction. Furthermore deficits in passive avoidance may indicate an inability to *inhibit* a response (that of going to the electrified food cup for food), and active avoidance requires the capacity to *initiate* a response.

The parameter of complexity has been further investigated. Brutowski et al (1960) trained dogs to associate one stimulus with approach (for food) and another for avoidance (for shock). After amygdalectomy they responded indiscriminately to both stimuli. They were thus unable to deal with two stimuli in one situation calling for discrimination between them and choice of the appropriate response. The important factor here might be either the complexity *per se*, or, as Weiskrantz has suggested, there was a defect in determining the reinforcement value of the stimulus, i.e. which stimulus 'meant' 'food' and which 'meant' 'pain'.

Schwartzbaum et al (1964) have further investigated the role of the amygdala in stimulus discrimination and generalization. They used an auditory tone of 550 c/s as the positive stimulus (reinforced with food—S^+) and a tone of 3,000 c/s remained unreinforced (S^-). Their animals after amygdalectomy showed a severe impairment of this discrimination (whereas ventral HC lesions had no effect). They gave their animals generalization tasks (in which the frequency range of both S^+ and S^- were both widened—to see what would still be recognized as a cue for food) and discrimination tasks where the frequencies of S^+ and S^- were brought closer together. In these tests the animals showed a disorder of function. They responded too often to the neutral stimulus and in the generalization task they made too many responses to tones between S^+ and S^-, and they required more sessions to regain criterion. The experimenters therefore supposed that the amygdala has a function in discriminating the reinforcing value of stimuli as well as merely recognizing the presence or absence of this.

Schwartzbaum (1960) has conducted some experiments to investigate further how the amygdala may be concerned with the reinforcing value of stimuli. Monkeys were trained to press a lever for food reward. Normally a monkey will press the lever more quickly to get a large food reward than it will to get a small one. Monkeys with amygdala lesions show much less of this modulation. They also eat too much and eat foods that normal monkeys will not eat. Therefore the amygdala may not only be necessary for determining the reinforcing value of single stimuli but also for the more subtle function of inter-relating different reinforcing stimuli: i.e. it enables an animal to respond to one set of events in relation to another. Such bilateral lesions do not have any effect on the spontaneous activity or inquisitive interest in the cat (Fernandez de Molina and Hunsperger, 1962). Schwartzbaum (1965) found that bilateral amygdala lesions in the monkey did not affect the postoperative learning of simple visual or somesthetic discriminations, but more complex tasks involving the inter-problem transfer of training were affected. The difficulties were in repressing responses to irrelevant features of the test object and in ceasing to make responses no longer adaptive. He sees the amygdala as selecting responses in terms of reinforcement contingencies.

Delgado (1964) has studied the effect of electrical stimulation of the amygdala on spontaneous behaviour in freely moving animals. For example, ten seconds' stimulation of the amygdala to a cat inhibited all alimentary conditioned reactions and the animal refused to eat for several days. Such stimulation can also induce such modulation of on-going behaviour as increasing the rate of chewing or the amount of time spent in play activity. The amygdala would appear then to modulate complex behaviour—in particular with respect to motivation, conditioning and reinforcement—much as the corpus striatum (of which it will be recalled that the amygdala is a specialized part) modulates the pattern of motor movements. The amygdala also plays some part in this latter function as stimulation of the lateral amygdala leads to facilitation of cortically induced movements whereas these can be inhibited by stimulation of its medial division.

One complication in interpreting these results is introduced by the fact that the corticomedial division of the amygdala is a positive reward centre for electrical self-stimulation using Olds's well-known technique. That is to say that a rat with electrodes implanted in this part of the brain will press a lever repeatedly to deliver a stimulus to his own brain. The basolateral division is a negative punishing area—that is a rat will press a lever to turn off a stimulus delivered to this region. It is therefore possible that stimulation of the amygdala during a learning trial may result in an apparent defect in learning that may really be due, not to any interference with the mechanisms of learning, but merely because the rat is attending to 'pleasureable' sensation, or intent on avoiding painful sensations, to the exclusion of attending to the learning task. This difficulty applies widely to all electrical stimulation studies since much of the limbic system is positive or negative in Olds's sense.

The possible role of emotional factors in confusing investigations into the role of the amygdala in learning is further illustrated by some experiments of Fonberg (1963). Dogs were trained to a CAR with the UCS either an electric shock to the skin or to the 'fear' centre of the hypothalamus. Stimulation of the basolateral division of the amygdala did not affect the CAR but it quietened the animals between trials. Those expecting hypothalamic stimulation were particularly frightened and restless. Stimulation of the amygdala abolished this fear and also the outbursts of fear and aggression induced by the actual stimulation of the hypothalamus. The animals were fully attentive during amygdala stimulation and could orient to new stimuli.

3.2.4 THE AMYGDALA AND ENDOCRINE FUNCTION

The amygdala has important connections with the pituitary–adrenal stress mechanism. Stimulation of the basolateral division activates this mechanism and HC stimulation inhibits it. Lesions of the amygdala delay the rise of plasma-free cortisone (PFC) in the blood following immobilization stress (the normal shows a 200 per cent rise in only 30 minutes: an amygdala lesion increases this time to 4 hours). The resting levels were normal. With HC lesions on the other hand there was a normal response to stress but the resting levels of PFC were significantly raised. The conclusion (see Knigge, 1961) was that the amygdala is needed for acute and rapid activation of the hypothalomo-hypophyseal system and that the HC contributes a tonic inhibitory influence on ACTH secretion. Electrical stimulation of the amygdala via indwelling electrodes in the conscious monkey produces marked acute elevations of plasma 17—OHCS levels (Rubin et al, 1966). HC stimulation (for only 90 minutes) produces a marked fall that may last for several days (Mason et al, 1961). Lesions of the amygdala and HC do not have much effect on pituitary gonadotropic or thyrotropic activity. Repeated stimulation of the medial nucleus and pyriform cortex, however, induced hypersexual behaviour and altered patterns of adrenocortical hormone excretion in female animals. This behaviour was not seen in ovariectomized animals (Lissák and Endröczi, 1961). It will be recalled that lesions of the pyriform cortex induce testosterone dependent hypersexuality in male animals. Possibly repeated stimulation of the pyriform cortex induces functional exhaustion or possibly this cortex has opposite functions in the two sexes. In any event the pyriform cortex would appear to be an important neuroendocrine centre. In amygdalectomized monkeys the GSR cannot be conditioned and it fails to show normal differential responses to different intensities of the S. The organism is thus less sensitive to 'nuances in stimulus characteristics' (Bagshaw and Coppock, 1968). In Goddard's view (1964) the function of the amygdala is to consolidate the association between a neutral stimulus and an aversive one. He found that continuous low-intensity stimulation of the amygdala (60 c/s) impairs fear-motivated learning but does not

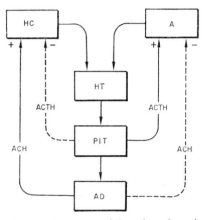

Figure 23.   Feedback control of the adrenal cortical secretion

HC	Hippocampus	AD	Adrenal
A	Amygdala	ACH	Adrenocortical hormone
HT	Hypothalamus	ACTH	Adrenocorticotrophic
PIT	Pituitary		hormone

affect food-motivated learning. However, the difficulty of making generalizations on the basis of electrical stimulation using limited stimulus parameters has been mentioned above.

The amygdala and HC are also involved in the higher control of ovarian function. Stimulation of the centromedian amygdala gives rise to ovulation and the HC theta rhythm increases some 30 per cent during oestrus. Stimulation of the dorsal HC gives rise to evoked potentials in the arcuate nucleus of the hypothalamus which leads in turn to stimulation of progesterone production by the ovary. ACTH depresses the HC theta and gives 40 c/s spindle bursts. Following ACTH the potentials evoked in the arcuate nucleus by HC stimulation are inhibited for 24 hours and the potentials evoked by stimulation of the amygdala are markedly potentiated. Kawakami et al (1967) have suggested the scheme shown in figure 23.

Fendler et al (1961) have confirmed that the HC exerts an inhibitory effect on the pituitary–adrenal system. They ablated the HC bilaterally in adult cats and tested them from 1 to 3 months later. They found a three-fold increase in blood corticoid levels as compared with normal cats and cats with neocortical ablations. There was no change in adrenal weight. Endröczi et al (1959) found a decrease in blood corticoids following HC stimulation. However, Endröczi and Lissák (1962) found that stimulation of the dorsal HC at low frequencies depressed the release of ACTH induced by painful stimulation whereas stimulation at higher frequencies had the opposite effect.

Stimulation of the amygdala (lateral, medial and basal nuclei) also induce release of antidiuretic hormone (Hayward and Smith, 1963). The response was rapid suggesting some direct neural pathway rather than an indirect response to some autonomic disturbance. They note that the amygdala is affected by vagal impulses. Stimulation of the other amygdaloid nuclei or of the pyriform cortex had no effect.

The effects of amygdalectomy may also depend in part on the age at which the operation was done. Bilateral lesions of the amygdala and pyriform cortex in 53-day-old kittens led to none of the behavioural reactions reported following this operation in older cats, in particular the immediately post-operative stage of semi-stupor (Kling, 1962). Neither did there occur any later development of growth deficit or hypopituitarism. In contrast Koikegami et al (1958) reported that the operation in infant animals causes panhypopituitarism, lack of growth and early death. Riss et al (1963) reported diminished gonadal and adrenal development following bilateral HC damage in 1-week-old rats. Bilateral pyriform lobe damage caused a precocious upsurge in running activity (normally seen at puberty) but no gonadal hypertrophy.

The cingulate gyrus also has an effect on this sytem. Bilateral coagulation in the rat leads to an increase of corticosteroid output (Bohus, 1961). Ibayashi et al (1963) claimed that stimulation of

E

the gyrus caused a rise in blood ACTH plus autonomic changes. As might be expected hypophysectomy prevented the rise in ACTH but not the autonomic changes. Adrenocortical hormones themselves have an effect on behaviour. If monkeys are treated with ACTH during the acquisition of a CAR they show less subsequent reaction to the CS and a very rapid rate of extinction of the CAR (Mirsky et al, 1953). They have been as it were protected from the disrupted effect of fear. Lissák and Endröczi (1961) report the same effect following the administration of cortisone. Dogs were conditioned to push a swing door to reach food on hearing a bell. When the reflex reaction was well established, on three successive days the dogs received an electric shock just after the bell sounded: then the bell was again sounded without shock on successive days. The CR was abolished, to return spontaneously after a few days. In general, those dogs that recovered quickly had low hydrocortisone/cortisone ratios in the adrenal vein blood whereas those dogs that took a long time to recover had high ratios. In another experiment using the same procedure half the animals were given hydrocortisone for a week before the shocks were given. They all showed much 'neurotic' reaction and took a long time to recover. Hydrocortisone in this case had the opposite effect from ACTH in Mirsky's experiment in potentiating the CAR and in speeding up the rate of extinction. In any case the role of the adrenocortical hormones and of ACTH in evaluating the effects of stimulation of the amygdala cannot be ignored.

Gunne and Reis (1963) linked changes in brain catecholamines with stimulation of the amygdala. They stimulated the amygdala (cat) for 3 minutes and repeated this every 5 minutes. At first they obtained the usual alerting responses with motor and autonomic effects and occasional hissing and growling. The cats were quiet in time off (the time free from stimulus). After a period of time that varied from 15 to 120 minutes clawing, hissing, snarling and attack resulted with some aggressive behaviour and autonomic responses in time off. At the end of 3 hours they obtained full-blown aggressive outbursts lasting well into time off. In these animals there was a marked increase in brain noradrenaline and adrenal adrenaline, a moderate increase in adrenal noradrenaline but no increase in brain dopamine. These measurements were carried out in the brainstem and the contralateral hemisphere. If no defence reaction occurred in reaction to amygdala stimulation, there were no changes in the brain catecholamines. The authors supposed that their results might indicate that the liberation of brain catecholamines was limited to noradrenaline or that a difference in the rate of resynthesis might be responsible.

In a series of pharmacological studies, Allikinets and Lapin (1967) showed that bilateral amygdala lesions in rats reduced the normal inhibitory effects of imipramine on exploratory behaviour; amphetamine had an increased stimulant action and LSD had less effect. The depressive actions of reserpine are increased and the initial excitatory phase absent. This indicates the involvement of adrenergic and perhaps serotoninergic mechanisms in amygdala action.

Killam and Killam (1967) have carried out a series of important experiments on the pharmacology of conditioning mechanisms. The stimulus was a series of geometrical shapes flickering at 10 c/s and the discrimination learning tasks were made progressively more difficult. Recordings were made from different loci in the brain. Evoked activity from the lateral geniculate body became progressively more complex as the discrimination became more difficult. The same was true for the amygdala and the 40 c/s rhythm became prominent with increasing difficulty of the task, possibly indicating increased anxiety. The effect of atropine was to increase the evoked 10 c/s rhythm in the HC and visual pathways and greatly to inhibit the 40 c/s rhythm in the amygdala. Reserpine augmented this rhythm, an effect reversed by amphetamine. Thus the amygdala rhythm would appear to be subject to dual control (cholinergic—excitatory; adrenergic—inhibitory).

3.2.5 HUMAN STUDIES

Stimulation of the amygdala in conscious human beings gives the following results:

(1) Various bodily and visceral sensations ('nausea', 'hot',

'chill', 'pins and needles', 'a shock', 'funny feeling', etc.). These are vague and hard to localize and can also be obtained by stimulation of the insula region. They indicate the extensive sensory inflow to the amygdala.

(2) Chewing movements.

(3) Various forms of mental confusion extending to a typical psychomotor epileptic seizure with complete unresponsiveness, confused speech and automatic behaviour with subsequent amnesia. These effects were only obtained, however, when seizure activity had propagated widely throughout the temporal lobe both in its cortical and subcortical portions. In patients with temporal lobe epilepsy electrical stimulation of the amygdala can lead to all the clinical features of their seizures (Chatrian and Chapman, 1960).

The clinical features of temporal lobe epilepsy reflect temporal lobe and amygdaloid function. This will be dealt with in more detail later but in this context the lowered rage threshold and outbursts of aggression suggest an upset in amygdala function. The interictal features of temporary lobe epilepsy—irritability, a tendency to sudden violent outbursts of rage, slow 'sticky' thinking, loss of libido and disturbances of appetite, can readily be understood in terms of chronic subictal stimulation of the amygdala.

Narabayashi et al (1963) have reported on a series of 60 patients, mainly children with temporal lobe epilepsy and severe behaviour disorders, who were treated with stereotactic amygdaloidectomy. The lateral nucleus was the target. The children were excitable, aggressive, irritable, destructive and showed an impairment in attention. The EEG from the amygdala commonly showed spikes and spindles. Following the operation (with was bilateral in 21 cases and unilateral in 39) there was a marked improvement in 29 cases, and a moderate improvement in 22. The children became calm, obedient and showed good social adjustment in spite of the fact that all but 6 showed some degree of mental defect. In no case were any of the other elements of the Klüver–Bucy syndrome induced and there was no disturbance of memory. This operation has also been carried out on aggressive psychotic patients (Green et al, 1951; Pool, 1954; Scoville, 1954). In the main a decrease in assaultive behaviour resulted but some patients showed organic mental deterioration and child-like behaviour and speech.

3.3 The role of the hippocampus

3.3.1 ANIMAL STUDIES

One major component of the Klüver–Bucy syndrome in man is the inability to lay down permanent memories. Destruction of permanent memory formation is also a feature of the Korsakoff syndrome where the lesions are located in the grey matter surrounding the IIIrd ventricle and aqueduct (including the limbic midbrain area), the mamillary bodies and the HC. What happens, then, when we carry out bilateral ablation of the HC in animals? In birds this leads to permanent loss of imprinting behaviour. In mammals there has been some conflict of opinion. Some workers claimed that retention of pre-operatively learned tasks is not interfered with (e.g. Yasukochi et al, 1962; Pribram and Weiskrantz, 1955; Lashley, quoted by Kaada et al, 1961). Some claimed the opposite (e.g. Kaada et al, 1961)—using rats and the CAR and maze learning. They claim that retention is interfered with only if pre-operative training was incomplete. Some have stated that HC ablations impair new learning (e.g. Moore, 1964; Buresova et al, 1962; Yasukochi et al, 1962; Thomas and Otis, 1958b) others that it does not (e.g. Allen, 1938, 1940). Isaacson and Wickelgren (1962) found that HC ablation impairs the rat's ability to make a passive avoidance response but it does not affect the ability to acquire active avoidance responses. Stepien et al (1960) noted that many so-called 'tests for recent memory' do not in fact test recent memory. So they tested monkeys using a test that they claimed does so—Konorski's compound stimuli test. In this Sx and Sy are two different stimuli—say tones of different pitch. The meaning of these stimuli is given by sounding one then the other. If they are the same (i.e. Sx followed by Sx, or Sy followed by Sy) this is positively rewarded (with food). If they are different (e.g. Sx followed by Sy or Sy followed by Sx) this is negatively rewarded (shock). The interval between Sx and Sy was 5 seconds.

Therefore the first stimulus *must* be remembered for 5 seconds if the animal is to learn the discrimination. The monkeys were then divided into three groups with removals of different parts: (i) the superior temporal gyrus (ii) the inferior temporal gyrus and (iii) uncus, HC, HC gyrus and amygdala. The first group showed a postoperative defect in auditory but not visual compound learning. The second group showed the reverse effect and the third group showed defects for both sensory modalities. The third group were then retested and it was established that (*a*) they were neither blind nor deaf; (*b*) they had no difficulty in learning tasks involving simple frequency discriminations and (*c*) they could learn new tasks involving delays of more than 5 seconds *provided that the meaning of the first stimulus does not depend on the second stimulus.* For example they could learn the following tasks:

(1) whistle–pause–buzzer–act; is punished
(2) buzzer–act;   is rewarded.

In this test the whistle does not have to be retained as such to compare with the buzzer as it gives the negative clue right away and the animal knows at once what to do when the buzzer is sounded later. That is to say there is no impairment of classical delayed learning and no loss of motivation. However, these animals could not relearn the compound stimuli task unless the time between the stimuli was reduced nearly to zero. Penfield found in humans that bilateral lesions of the HC caused a recent memory defect for both verbal and non-verbal material—with no change in attention, concentration, reasoning ability, intelligence, vocabulary or professional skills. The patients could all retain in mind a sentence or short sequence of numbers for up to 15 minutes, if they were permitted to keep them in mind the entire time— i.e. if they were instructed to do so and were protected from any distractions. If their attention wandered for 1 second all was lost. The neocortex of, and surrounding, the primary sensory areas are concerned in *immediate* memory for that particular modality.

Karmos and Grastyán (1962) tested cats with bilateral HC lesions. In their spontaneous behaviour they noted that the cats were generally overactive and showed very strong orienting responses. In the simple type of sound–food reflex there was no change in retention of old learning or establishment of new learning. But the orienting reflex was not inhibited early in the learning process as it is in normal cats. When the buzzer sounded a well-trained cat went straight to the food box. The HC cat went to the loudspeaker, sniffed at it, stood up to face it and then performed long-lasting searching movements until it saw the food box by chance when it would go over to it. Thus the animal eventually succeeded in the task but the reaction time was both longer and more variable than in normal animals. If a delayed reaction test is tried where the buzzer sounds over one of three boxes but the animal is not released until 1 minute later, normal cats can learn which box to go to in 7–13 days, HC cats never. As soon as the buzzer sounded they showed an exaggerated orienting response, then general excitement and a complete failure to go to the correct box. Thus the HC animal reacts by a hyperactive orienting response which can only be inhibited with difficulty, and, in this more *complex* task of recent memory, it fails. The relationship of the HC to the orienting response will be discussed further below (chapter 5).

The type of conditioned response may also be important. For example is it a response where emotion is involved or only a simple movement response? The Walter Reed group (Brady, 1958) found that HC lesions eliminate the conditioned fear response (CFR) and make it almost impossible to recondition them.

In a recent comprehensive review Douglas (1967) has examined the role of the HC in memory formation and has cast doubt on several previous notions in this field, and in particular has pointed to the apparent contradictions between human and animal studies. The memory deficit produced in humans by HC lesions has been described by clinicians as a 'loss of recent memory' when it is really the failure to lay down permanent memories. This could be due to interference with a number of possible mechanisms. For example, the HC may be needed to protect memory traces from disruption by the ceaseless stream of sensory impulses during a crucial phase of consolidation. However, many of the previous tasks that were thought to measure memory, did not in fact do so, and much confusion has resulted in the literature. In particular the hypothesis has gained ground that the HC may be involved in the suppression of unwanted previously learned responses. As mentioned above lesions of the HC and septum produce a deficit of passive avoidance but none of active avoidance. Cingulate lesions have the opposite effect. In order to measure 'passive avoidance' the usual procedure is to electrify the food box, so that the animal receives an electric shock when it tries to feed. Thus in order to avoid the shock it has to inhibit its tendency to approach the box for food. In active avoidance the animal merely has to jump onto a safe platform when it hears the CS signalling the imminence of shock applied to the grid floor of the cage. HC rats are very resistant to the extinction of a conditioned response and this too requires the inhibition of a previously learned response. Further evidence for this hypothesis is provided by the following facts: HC lesions (i) prevent reversal learning (ii) lead to a deterioration of performance in multiple choice mazes (iii) produce an inability to make alternate responses to two S (iv) produce a deficiency in sequential discrimination tasks and (v) inhibit the conditioned emotional response. This response is obtained as follows. A rat is trained to press a lever for food reward. It is then further conditioned to a sound–shock sequence. If the buzzer is then sounded while the rat is pressing the lever for food, the latter activity stops and the rat crouches down and shows the behavioural signs of fear. In all these the rat has to inhibit a learned response that was previously adaptive to the situation but is no longer so. It has repeatedly been demonstrated that HC animals do better in tasks in which a disruptive inhibitory tendency is present (as in the two-way shuttle box) and they do worse if inhibition is required (as in the CER). No differences are observed in tasks where no inhibition is involved at all. HC lesions impair the inhibition only of learned behaviour and not of unlearned responses such as exploratory behaviour (Kimble et al, 1966). However, the matter is not that simple. In Konorski's test reported above, subsequent analysis showed that the failure of the HC animals in the test was due almost entirely to errors of commission and not to errors of omission. That is the animals responded to too many negative signals($S_x \ldots S_y$) and did not miss any positive ones ($S_x \ldots S_x$): thus it appeared they could not suppress the unwanted response. Therefore, in order to measure this type of memory properly, a task must be employed that does not involve inhibition. Such a test was used by Correll and Scoville (1965)—the delayed matching test. In this a coloured thread is shown and then some seconds later, two threads, and the monkey is rewarded for touching the matching colour. HC lesions do not affect performance of this test. Therefore, Douglas concludes, the connection between the HC and memory is not proven and he makes the following hypothesis. The normal process of memory storage may be much more complex than the simple imprinting of an engram on a collection of neurones. The HC may be involved in integrating processed central representations of the S with items recalled from the permanent memory store. The HC may be concerned with sorting the sensory input for items of relevance. Thus the HC animals cannot withhold a response because they cannot categorize response inducing stimuli. Human memory defects following HC lesions may also be due to disruption of the normal process of sorting, categorization and organization of stimuli. Meissner (1968) has also suggested that laying down permanent memory is a most complex process involving a coding and integrating mechanism which requires the function of sequential organization. These concepts will be discussed further in chapters 5 and 6.

Wickelgren and Isaacson (1963) trained rats on a simple runway. Latencies (i.e. the time before they set off to run down the course) and the running times decreased day by day. Then on the 8th and 9th days a new but totally irrelevant stimulus was introduced in the form of a step at the entrance of the runway. With this the latency of the normal rats immediately rose. They waited presumably to take stock of this new feature in the previously familiar environment. Rats with bilateral HC lesions did not do so. They also had consistently shorter latencies. They seemed less concerned with novel features in their environment. The experimenters therefore suggested that the HC may be concerned with the ability to respond correctly to novel stimuli.

Further support for the hypothesis that the function of the HC is to categorize sensory information has come fron Winocur and Salzen (1968). They carried out a series of experiments using different-sized circles as S. They found no deficit in ordinary retention and acquisition tasks in HC animals, but as soon as stimuli negative before operation were made positive after the operation, the HC animals did badly. However, the precise details of the S changes were a significant variable and the authors felt that no general perseverative tendency was present but rather a more complex reaction. In the transfer tasks the rats responded by an initial exploration and random responses typical of animals faced with an entirely new task. Thus they felt that the HC rats were unable to categorize new sensory information. Stein and Kimble (1966), note that rats in a maze cannot habituate to irrelevant stimuli and so learn slowly. They suggest that HC animals '. . . cannot distinguish as rapidly between information which has been scanned previously and is judged redundant or irrelevant and that which is critical for adequate performance'.

Further support for the hypothesis that the HC is needed to inhibit a previously learned response was provided by Webster and Voneida (1964) in their studies of reversal learning in cats; by Kimble and Kimble (1965) using rats and a Y maze; and by Clark and Isaacson (1965) using rats and a DRL schedule.

Swanson and Isaacson (1967) have suggested, on the basis of operant conditioning experiments, that the apparent inability to withhold a response following HC lesions is not a 'motor' phenomenon, but is really due to the lack of the normal dampening effect of the HC on the frustration reaction. Likewise Rabe and Haddad (1968) examined the performance of HC rats using a Fixed Ratio operant conditioning schedule. They found the marked resistance to extinction already reported by many workers and felt that their results indicated that behaviour was disrupted by increased emotional frustration (to delay of anticipated reward) rather than motor perseveration. HC lesions do not produce an abnormal perseveration to every S—for example it actually reduces perseveration of the freezing response to a noxious stimulus. Furthermore approach behaviour was only potentiated in rats in specific 'interesting' environments (Kaplan, 1968). Once involved in goal-directed behaviour HC rats are less distractible by other S. Thus Kaplan suggests that the HC may be involved in the motivational aspects of stimuli. Kambach (1967) conducted an experiment designed to test whether HC lesions impair habituation to novel S or the ability to withold a response. Rats were placed in a two-lever Skinner box. A press on lever 1 diminished the lighting of the box for a period. A press on lever 2 had no effect. Normally rats will press lever 1 for about $\frac{1}{2}$ hour and will then habituate. HC rats, when satiated, made more presses than satiated controls and did not habituate. Thus food-satiated HC rats behaved just like food-deprived control rats (and deprived HC rats behaved rather like deprived controls). Kambach suggests that '. . . the hippocampus may be functionally involved in the mediation of motivational behavior, possibly by biasing the animal's rate of habituation to novel stimuli as a function of the motivational state of the animal'.

Grossman and Mountford (1964) used functional ablations of the HC obtained by local injection of KCl. They doubt whether the HC really affects either the acquisition or the retention of memories and suggest instead that it may be concerned with motivation. The number of correct choices in a simple black–white discrimination test in a T maze was not affected by HC lesions. However, the level of performance was definitely affected in that the animals failed to respond to the CS as quickly, approached the choice point more slowly, took more time to make their decision and their extinction rate was increased. All this could be explained on the basis of a low motivational state.

However, several workers have come to the defence of the hypothesis that the HC does, after all, play a role in memory formation. Thompson et al (1964) made rats learn a simple maze where the correct side to go was alternated every day. If there was a 30-second period between trials, the HC rats learned normally, but they did not do so if the delay was increased to 30 minutes. Drachman and Ommaya (1964) also point out the discrepancy between human and animal studies in the role assigned to the HC in memory formation. This is partly due to different meaning of the term. In animal work 'short term memory' means 'transient memory decaying with time and leaving no permanent trace'. In human work it is used loosely to cover the recollection of a memorandum for a short period. Recent memory loss in humans depends more on the complexity of the memorandum than on the passage of time. They argue that what has been interpreted as 'impaired recent memory' in humans corresponds to impaired acquisition and storage in animals. In a later paper Drachman and Arbit (1966) report the result of testing five patients with bilateral HC lesions, who showed memory deficits. Their digit span was normal (i.e. for digits presented only once) but their total digit storage capacity (for digits repeated up to 20 times) was only 8·6 as compared with the normal 20. They did not show any excess perseveration. They also showed a retrograde amnesia, usually incomplete, lasting for from a few days to a few years. The authors suggest that the HC is essential for the permanent storage of new memories and may act as a temporary storage depot for engrams carrying the new memory. 'Short-term memory' they define as dealing only with '. . . subspan memoranda, evanescently, as long as the subject's attention is directed towards the memorandum'. 'Long-term memory' (storage) deals with '. . . supraspan memoranda held for long and short intervals and with subspan memoranda recalled following the redirection of attention'.

In *stimulation studies* complications are introduced by the fact that epileptic activity is readily evoked in the HC and propagates to other parts of the brain including the RF, amygdala and temporal neocortex. When this happens a cataleptic state is induced which will interfere with any test for learning. The other complications from all stimulation studies of the limbic system that we have already discussed also apply. Green (1964) has argued that stimulation and ablation studies as ordinarily performed are untrustworthy and should be replaced by reversible lesions (e.g. local cooling or injection of procaine). However, this in turn raises the problem of the verification of the actual location of injection. The usual contradictions are in evidence. Some workers claim that HC stimulation affects mainly rates of extinction (Correll, 1957). Others claim that this depresses both CAR and approach reactions and that this is associated with cortical slow waves as in behavioural extinction. Thus Lissák supposes that the HC has a specific inhibitory effect on the RF. HC stimulation seems to have little effect on simple bar-pressing for food reward (Knott et al, 1960). In freely moving animals, it causes arrest and bewilderment but only if after-discharges have been provoked and presumably, as in the case of the amygdala, widespread epileptic activity. Endröczi and Lissák (1962), however, claim that HC stimulation blocks spontaneous activity and the performance of alimentary CRs. In the cat in which attack behaviour is induced by stimulation of the hypothalamus, simultaneous stimulation of the ventral HC shortens the latency to attack whereas stimulation of the dorsal HC has the opposite effect (Siegal and Flynn, 1968). In humans Brazier (1964) states that *bilateral* HC stimulation leads to transient and reversible loss of memory function without apparent impairment of other faculties.

Other alleged aspects of HC function besides recent memory have been investigated.

Ellen and Powell (1962) investigated the hypothesis that the HC is concerned with temporal discrimination. They used 4 groups of 6 rats each—controls, with septal lesions, with unilateral HC lesions and with bilateral HC lesions. The task was a fixed interval (FI) food reward schedule. In this the animal must press a lever and the food reward comes at fixed intervals—say once a minute—provided that the animal has pressed the lever at least once during the preceding minute. Under these circumstances a normal animal learns to wait until the minute is almost up and then it will press the lever repeatedly until the food reward is obtained and then stop. In the rats with HC lesions (1) there were no such changes at these different times suggesting a failure of 'temporal discrimination': (2) they also pressed the lever less often in the last 10 seconds of the FI schedule, suggesting, to the experimenters, a 'decline in motivation' and (3) they did not learn to stop pressing the lever immediately after the food reward—suggesting a failure to inhibit an environmentally irrelevant response or perseveration of an old response. However, it would seem that findings (2) and (3) logically follow from (1) and they may furthermore merely reflect in whole or in part loss of recent memory in a complex situation.

Pribram's theory of HC function suggests that it may be concerned with the organization of complex behaviour sequences. Kimble and Pribram (1963) tested this hypothesis as follows. Eight monkeys were trained in a simple discrimination task (to distinguish between the figures 6 and 4) for food reward. Then four of these monkeys were subjected to bilateral HC ablations and all were again tested on this task. The operated monkeys showed no deficit. Both groups were given a more difficult task to learn. They were faced with 16 panels of numbers, two of which were 1s. The task was to learn to press both 1s in either order. Normal monkeys managed this in an average of 298 trials; three HC monkeys failed to learn in 1,200 trials but one succeeded in 130. The next task was to learn to press 1 and then 5 in that order. This the normals learned in an average of 1,216 trials but HC monkeys took 1,897 (p <0·01 for the difference). The authors suggest that this result could not be due to any simple memory defect as HC ablations had no effect on simple discriminations even if 6 minutes were allowed to elapse between presentations of the two members of the pair of stimuli to be discriminated. They suggest that '. . . bilateral hippocampal lesions interfere selectively with the acquisition of behaviours which involve the execution of sequential responses.'

Ellen and Powell (1963), however, showed that the zona incerta, rather than the HC or septum, played a role in timing behaviour. Rats with lesions of the zona incerta did not show the usual scalloping on FI schedules of reinforcement. Lesions of the HC and septum did not produce this effect. Previous reports that lesions of the mamillary bodies induce this effect were probably due to concomitant damage to the zona incerta.

Webster and Voneida (1964) have investigated the effect of HC lesions on cats with 'split-brain' preparations. In these the corpus callosum is cut and each half of the cerebrum functions independently as far as learning sensory discrimination is concerned. For example, a sensory discrimination learned with one paw, is not 'available' to the other paw. One hemisphere can thus act as a control for a lesion placed in the other. These authors made lesions in one HC in the 'split-brain' cats, without damage to amygdala or entorhinal area. They then trained the animals in a tactile sensory discrimination task where a cat has to learn to depress one of two levers solely on a basis of tactile clues ('rough' v. 'smooth', 'vertical wooden bars' v. 'horizontal bars', etc.). The paw that could be used was controlled by the geometry of the box.

They found that there was no difference between the normal hemisphere and the 'HC hemisphere' in the *acquisition* of learning of the discrimination response. The cats were next tested on reversal learning. In this the cat is trained to associate one lever with 'food' and the other with 'no food'. Then the levers are simply reversed and the number of trials counted for the cat to learn to press the new 'food' lever. This naturally requires suppression of the previous response as this was previously the 'no food' lever. In this case, removal of the HC had a marked effect and the 'HC hemisphere' took between 2 and 6 times as long to acquire the reverse habit as did the normal hemisphere. Similarly, an animal with a unilateral HC lesion and intact commissures transferred learning normally (i.e. what was learnt with one paw was available to the other) and showed normal reversal learning. If the other HC was now ablated, the reversal learning was severely impaired.

Then two further tests were run. In the *extinction of response* measure there was no food reinforcement whichever lever was pressed. HC lesions had no effect on the rate of this extinction. In the *extinction of discrimination* measure a press on either lever is rewarded with food. In the case of the normal hemisphere the animal presses either lever equally after only 1 day on this schedule. The HC hemisphere is highly resistant to this discrimination and the animal continued to press preferentially the old '+' lever for 6–20+ days. (This is confirmed by Porter et al, 1964.)

The authors, therefore, concluded that the HC is not necessary for acquiring a single response based on a sensory discrimination but that it is necessary if a previously learned response has to be extinguished in the process. HC lesions have been reported to induce grave deficiencies of maternal behaviour in the rat (Kimble et al, 1967). The mothers were poor nest-builders, and showed poor hover (nursing) behaviour and poor retrieval rates. More time was spent in exploration. There was no evidence of any active avoidance of the pups, and cannibalism occurred.

The HC also seems to be concerned in the response to painful stimuli. A mild painful S gives simple RF and cortical arousal but a strong one gives marked HC theta together with the behavioural reaction of crying and biting the electrodes (Soulairac et al, 1967). Morphine and similar analgesics specifically prevent this HC reaction and have no effect on the RF. The startle and escape reaction seems to be mediated by the RF and the crying, biting reaction by the HC. Midbrain lesions and dibenamine depress the former and potentiate the latter whereas amphetamine, eserine and atropine have the opposite effect.

The HC receives both noradrenergic and cholinergic innervation (Grant and Jarrard, 1968). These workers injected drug crystals into various loci. NE had only a slight effect on the HC. It increased eating and led to some hoarding for some 10 minutes. Carbachol had a much more potent action. In the anterior dorsal area it led to a marked increase in drinking for 20–40 minutes with some increase in general activity. In the posterior HC it increased eating and the animals became very alert and moved excitedly about the cage. In some seizures were induced.

3.3.2 HUMAN STUDIES

We have noted that bilateral removal of the HC in man leads to severe and permanent loss of the ability to lay down permanent memory. A short sentence or list of numbers can be remembered as long as it is kept continually in mind but as soon as attention wavers, the memory is lost. Victor et al (1961) have reported on a human case with thrombosis of both posterior cerebral arteries leading to degeneration of HC, fornix and mamillary bodies. The amygdala and uncus were unaffected. The patient showed a gross memory defect and an inability to learn or retain new facts and skills. He showed a retrograde amnesia for $2\frac{1}{2}$ years prior to his stroke but his memory for earlier events was unimpaired. These authors note that the neurofibrillary changes of Alzheimer's disease, where profound early memory loss is a prominent feature, is particularly marked in the HC. Some cases of inclusion cell encephalitis affect particularly the inferomedial portion of the temporal lobe and can lead to a pure memory loss.

The role of the mamillary bodies is more obscure. The pathological lesions of Korsakoff's syndrome affect these bodies markedly but they also affect the grey matter surrounding the IIIrd ventricle and the aqueduct and the dorsomedial nucleus of the thalamus. Bilateral lesions of this latter nucleus in humans leads to temporary disorientation and memory defect (q.v.) But these effects may be nonspecific as similar temporary changes may follow on other brain operations (e.g. stereotactic operations on the basal ganglia in Parkinsonism). Cutting the anterior pillar of the fornix on both sides in man leads to no disturbance of memory (Barbizet, 1963)—although the multiple pathways typical of limbic connections may account for results such as this. It is possible that the lesions in the limbic area of the midbrain in Korsakoff's syndrome are as important as those in the mamillary bodies if not more so. The ability to lay down permanent memory depends certainly on the integrity of the HC and possibly more on the integrity of the circuit HC–limbic area of midbrain–intralaminar thalamic nuclei–HC than on the classical Papez circuit. *Immediate* memory (that which we can remember if we do not take our attention from it) does not depend apparently on the HC and may be a function of primary sensory cortex and parasensory cortex.

3.4 The role of the septum

It has been suggested that the septum may function as the most rostral portion of the reticular activating system. This has a portion in the medulla and pons, a mesencephalic portion in the midbrain, a diencephalic portion in the form of the intralaminar and midline thalamic nuclei and perhaps a telencephalic portion —the septum—derived from the anterior part of the most medial portion of the cerebral vesicles close to the interventricular foramen. This may explain the important role of the septum in HC arousal. A septal lesion will block the theta rhythm in the HC following an alerting stimulus and stimulation of the septum gives rise to large potentials in the HC. Petsche et al (1962) recorded from individual septal neurones as well as taking the HC EEG in the rabbit. They found two types of unit in the septum: A units that fired at random and B units that fired in synchrony with the HC theta rhythm. The B cell burst activity continued even if the HC rhythm changed suggesting that the former drove the latter and not the other way round.

Thus the septum has close functional, as well as two-way anatomical, connections with the HC and its appears to be an important station on the activation/inhibition pathway from the RF to the HC. Further details of this will be dealt with in chapter 4. The septum may also mediate neocortical–RF pathways.

Spiegel et al (1940) reported the production of sham rage following bilateral septal lesions and work by the Walter Reed group (Brady, 1958) showed that these lesions increase emotionality and potentiate the startle response (this is the response to an alarming S and should be differentiated from the arousal or alerting response which is evoked by an interesting S whose meaning is already known). These effects were only transient and were also seen after lesions of the HC. The role of the septum in suppressing undue emotionality is thus probably mediated by the HC. This finding has been confirmed by King (1958) who concludes that the septal region exerts a calming effect on behaviour, possibly by inhibiting the pituitary–adrenal stress mechanism. Septal coagulation leads to a rise of blood corticoids. The time course of this excess emotionality is the same as the duration of absence of the HC theta rhythm. This excessive emotionality is eliminated by the superimposition of a lesion in the amygdala. The septal–HC system inhibits ACTH release (Knigge and Hays, 1963).

Kaada et al (1962) claim that septal lesions like HC lesions render the animal incapable of inhibiting certain responses (like the approach response to the electrified food tray in the passive avoidance response). They note that stimulation of the subcallosal region can strongly inhibit on-going activity. The effects of septal lesions on learning are complicated, in the case of maze-learning, by the fact that exploratory behaviour becomes much more evident. Furthermore Endröczi and Lissák (1962) report that septal stimulation at 0·8 V leads to complete inhibition of all spontaneous motor activity but if a voltage of 2·0–4·0 is applied a powerful orientation response ensues which effectively interferes with CR performance. In the case of the CAR, septal lesions appear to improve acquisition in the rat (Thomas et al, 1959; King, 1958) but depress CAR retention and CER learning (Moore, 1964). The latter effect did not seem to correlate with the irritability syndrome seen in some of these septal cats. Ablation of the septum has been reported to abolish lever pressing to avoid pain but not lever pressing to gain food (Thomas et al, 1959).

The effect of septal stimulation is also complicated by the fact that this region (particularly its basomedial portion) constitutes a powerful reward area of self-stimulation. Stimulation higher in the septum produces arrest of all behaviour followed by a 're-bound' period after the end of the stimulation during which the animal appears afraid of harmless objects. Septal stimulation can also induce sleep, or loss of interest in food (to the extent of causing the animal to spit the food out and to make grimaces of distaste) and HC seizures.

Ellen et al (1964) have investigated the effect of septal lesions on rat DRL (differential reinforcement of low response rate) behaviour. In this only those responses are reinforced that occur at a fixed time interval (e.g. 20 seconds) following the previous response. Their previous work had shown that lesions of the septum, HC and mamillary body do not impair FI (fixed interval) reinforcement behaviour (in which the rat learns to press the lever every x seconds for food reward). The experimenters were seeking some neural mechanism for timing response and their negative results with the FI schedule led them to suppose that this might be too simple a task. So they chose the more complex DRL schedule. HC, hippocampal gyrus and callosal lesions had no effect on this response. The animals learned as do normals to space out their responses to give a modal inter-response time of about 20 seconds. Rats with septal lesions did not do this, however. From the beginning they showed a much higher rate of lever press and this did come down but not enough to succeed in gaining many rewards. The experimenters surmised that the septum may be necessary for inhibition of a response for an appreciable length of time. It is also, of course, possible that their results are due merely to emotional contamination—i.e. that this is a feature of the general irritable emotional state of animals with septal lesions. It may also be due in part to a more general interference with motor behaviour. They present evidence to suggest that this 'inhibitory influence' is mediated via the Papez circuit.

Schwartzbaum et al (1967) caution against trying to deduce *the* function of the septum from ablation and stimulation studies. The observed effects of septal lesions generally agreed on are: (i) depression of passive avoidance responses (ii) improvement of two-way shuttle box avoidance responses (iii) inhibition of the freezing response and increased emotionality (iv) increase in exploratory behaviour and (v) increase in general activity. Items (i) and (ii) are often explained on the basis of item (iii) but the further data of Schwartzbaum et al (1967) indicate that the phenomenon is too complex for any such simple explanation. In particular they found that general activity was *increased* in dim light in septal rats and the freezing responses were *potentiated* in bright light. These two findings account for much of the confusion in the literature. They felt that '. . . the effects of septal lesions on avoidance and activity reflect *in part* some common mode of dysfunction that is intimately tied to the reduced incidence of freezing responses', but that other factors to be considered in *any* behavioural response following septal lesions are hyperemotionality, reduction of fear, enhanced exploratory drive and lowered inhibitory control of the RF. Likewise the septum may not be *primarily* concerned with 'emotional' behaviour, but it may be involved in inhibitory control of the sensory input, motivation mechanisms, evaluation of reinforcement contingencies or in response inhibition, in close correlation with the HC (Schwartzbaum and Gay, 1966; Douglas and Raphelson, 1966; Burkett and Bunnell, 1966; Nielson et al,

1965; Schwartzbaum et al, 1964). The effects of septal lesions are differentially affected by lesions elsewhere. For example the hyper-reactivity and changes in freezing behaviour are abolished by a subsequent lesion in the amygdala (suggesting that they are due to unbalanced activity of the amygdala) whereas the depression of response inhibition is not so affected, and is probably linked to the HC (Schwartzbaum and Gay, 1966). Grossman (1964) showed that cholinergic stimulation of the medial septal area of the rat increased drinking but depressed eating and CAR behaviour. Cholinergic blocking agents had the opposite effects. Adrenergic agents potentiated the CAR and had no effect on food or water intake. Grossman suggested that a strong stimulus to one central motivation system may produce a secondary inhibition of other motivational systems. However, the septum is not merely an appendage of the HC. Electrical stimulation of the septum and the HC can act as CS for food reward and the rat can distinguish clearly between them (Ellen and Powell, 1966). In fact there is almost no generalization of this kind between subcortical structures (Nielson et al, 1962).

Lesions of the septal region in humans have been reported by Jefferson (1958) to produce coma similar to that following lesions of the midbrain portion of the RF. A similar akinetic state has been reported by Bond et al (1957) following lesions of the posterior septum, fornix and anterior thalamus. In humans again Zeman and King (1958) report on four cases of tumours of the septum pellucidum and adjacent structures. Early symptoms were very like the 'septal syndrome' of rats—i.e. emotional irritability with outbursts of aggression and uncontrolled emotion. The patients were also very sensitive to sudden noises. They also showed some memory defect. Later the general signs of an intracranial tumour intervened. The authors followed up these observations by injecting sarcoma cells into the septal region of five rats. In one the transplant was successful producing a small tumour in the anterior septum. This rat, and this rat alone, became vicious, fearful and unmanageable.

Thus many septal functions seem to be mediated by its close functional relationship with the HC. It may be concerned with consciousness and sleep, with the control of emotionality (perhaps indirectly through the inhibitory action of the HC on the stress mechanism) and with arousal/inhibitory relationships between the RF and the HC.

3.5 The role of the hypothalamus

This section will be concerned with the 'higher' functions of the hypothalamus in emotion, memory and the control of behaviour, and not with its purely vegetative functions considered in isolation nor with its various homeostatic functions in feeding, temperature control, etc. that have already been reviewed adequately elsewhere at length.

The classical studies of the role of the hypothalamus in behaviour were carried out by Hess. He divided it into two parts, the *ergotrophic* and the *trophotropic*. The former comprised the posterior hypothalamus (spreading over into the anterior midbrain area) and is associated with the sympathetic system. The trophotropic division is concerned with the parasympathetic system and has a scattered representation throughout the rest of the hypothalamus and outside it to include parts of the preoptic area and septum. Stimulation of the lateral hypothalamus (as well as the preoptic area, basal septal nuclei and basal medial thalamus) gives sham rage responses, whereas stimulation of the ergotrophic region gives escape behaviour.

Small lesions in the ventromedial hypothalamic nuclei produce very savage cats (Wheatley, 1944). These give well-calculated and well-directed aggressive reactions—i.e. real rage and not sham rage. This may be due to the unbalanced activity of the lateral hypothalamus. Egger and Flynn (1963) showed that electrical stimulation of the lateral hypothalamus led to effective attack behaviour. However, the attack behaviour elicited is still to some extent under environmental control. For example, the cat will attack a live rat more enthusiastically than a dead one and it will not attack a block of foam rubber the same size as a rat (Levison and Flynn, 1965). Delgado (1964) reports that stimulation of the lateral hypothalamus produces real rage whereas stimulation of the anterior hypothalamus produces sham rage—a mere motor display in which the animal will not even fight back if attacked. Stimulation in this anterior region also leads to adynamia and this may inhibit the direction of the rage attack. It should be noted that animals with all brain tissue above the hypothalamus removed are still capable of emotional and affective expression (Bromiley, 1948). The reflex support of the sham rage reaction depends on the activity of the RF. Sham rage can be produced by stimulation of the lateral RF and inhibited by stimulation of the medial RF (medial reticular and raphe nuclei only). Stimulation in the latter location during quiet periods has no observable effects (Bizzi et al, 1963). During the sham rage reaction produced by a section through the upper brain stem, the NE levels in the lower brain stem fall sharply. There is no change in levels of 5HT. The sham rage reaction produced by stimulation of the hypothalamus has the same effect. Lesions and stimuli in these areas that do not induce sham rage do not change NE levels. Therefore the activation of brain NE neurones may be important for the sham rage effect (Reis and Fuxe, 1968). The 'dual centre' theory of Anand and Brobeck (1951) suggests that the lateral hypothalamus is a 'feeding centre' which initiates feeding behaviour in response to olfactory and visual stimuli, and that the medial hypothalamus is a 'satiety centre', which inhibits the feeding centre when the animal is satiated. Following lesions to the lateral hypothalamus rats do not eat for many days. Rodgers et al (1965) tested whether this was due to a motor failure or a motivational deficit and concluded that the latter was the case—rats with these lesions can eat but do not do so because they are not hungry. Coons et al (1965) showed that stimulation of the lateral hypothalamus induced eating in the satiated animal and that the effect was not due to a non-specific facilitation of a dominant habit. Such stimulation also decreases the approach time to food in both conditioned and unconditioned behaviour and increases intestinal motility (Folkow and Rubinstein, 1966).

However, serious criticisms of much of the previous work on brain stimulation has come from Donovan (1966), Valenstein (1968), and Valenstein et al (1968). The former pointed out that many of these studies have used stainless steel electrodes which produce a surrounding irritative lesion due to the migration of Fe^{++} ions. This does not occur if platinum electrodes or radio-frequency coagulation are used. For example, the well-known effects of coagulation of the ventromedial nucleus of the hypothalamus (viciousness and hyperphagia) are seen only if steel electrodes are used and not in the case of radiofrequency coagulation. Thus the effect may be due to the irritation produced by the Fe^{++} ions in the ventrolateral area. Likewise lesions produced by platinum electrodes in the anterior hypothalamus of the infant rat induce early puberty by increasing gonadotrophin release. Electrolytic lesions of the amygdala do the same but surgical removal of the amygdala does not. Thus the effect may have been due to the migration of Fe^{++} ions to neighbouring areas. Donovan concludes that there is no valid evidence that individual nuclei control individual functions of the hypothalamus. Rubin (1968) has also shown that radiofrequency lesions of the ventromedial nucleus of the hypothalamus do not cause hyperphagia. Tungsten electrodes act just like steel ones. Thus considerable doubt has been cast on the existence of the medial 'satiation' centre. Moreover stimulation in exactly the same place with exactly the same stimulus parameters in the hypothalamus will evoke drinking, eating or gnawing depending on whether water, food or a lump of wood is present. This casts doubt on whether there really are specific 'eating' or 'drinking' circuits in the brain. Lesions in widespread areas (e.g. dorsomedial nucleus of the thalamus, temporal lobe cortex, amygdala and midbrain) can induce changes in feeding behaviour (Ehrlich, 1964).

The effect of lesions in the lateral hypothalamic area (depressing bar pressing for food) cannot be produced by sectioning the MFB rostral *or* caudal to the hypothalamus *or* the periventricular fibre system. The system has much redundancy and only lesions of the MFB rostral and caudal to the lateral hypothalamus are effective (Dicara and Wolf, 1968).

In humans a wide variety of affective responses have been reported following stimulation, operation, tumour, trauma, vascular lesions, infections, etc. involving the hypothalamus. Thus primitively organized and relatively undifferentiated patterns of behaviour can be organized by the hypothalamus and RF. These patterns are elaborated and integrated by the extensive limbic connections of the hypothalamus and these in turn mediate neocortical control. The hypothalamus may be concerned with reorganizing, recoding and redistributing instructions received from the HC and amygdala in terms of 'fight', 'flee', 'eat', 'approach', etc. into the appropriate sympathetic and parasympathetic concomitants of such behaviour. There is, it will be recalled, no sympathetic/parasympathetic differentiation in the higher limbic centres.

Unit recordings made by Murphy et al (1968) showed that the ventromedial nucleus is the main recipient of projections from the amygdala (both basal and lateral divisions) and the septum. These areas also project to the dorsal and lateral hypothalamic regions, but these areas receive most of their input from the midbrain tegmental region. Cells in the hypothalamus can be conditioned (Kamikawa et al, 1964). In these experiments the CS was a flash of light and the UCS a shock to the sciatic nerve. The conditioning was rather slow and usually required about 50 pairings of the stimuli.

The hypothalamus also plays an important role in learning. Partial destruction of the hypothalamus and RF can abolish an alimentary CR leaving the UCR intact (Gastaut, 1958). Lesions of the lateral hypothalamus interfere with visual and kinaesthetic learning; lesions of the posterior hypothalamus only with the latter. Lesions in the neighbourhood of the mamillary bodies interfere with learning a CAR and perhaps with its retention. Knott et al (1960), report that pre-mamillary lesions impair retention of an operant food-rewarded task: Dahl et al (1962), however, reported that this lesion had no effect on the retention of a CAR. It may often be the case that emotional changes contaminate learning. For example, Knott et al (1960) found that lesions in the pre-mamillary area impaired retention without producing any affective change whereas lesions in the ventromedial nucleus impaired 'learning' by reason of the increased savagery of the cats. The role of the mamillary bodies themselves is unclear.

Thompson and Hawkins (1961) have reported that, whereas lesions of the lateral hypothalamic area disrupt the visual CAR and discriminative learning, lesions of the mamillary bodies had no such effect. Posterior hypothalamic lesions merely made the cats savage. Kaada et al (1962) include the hypothalamus in the brain regions damage to which impairs the passive avoidance response.

Hypothalamic stimulation can lead to the abolition of new learning capacity. This may in part be due to competitive emotional responses, for much of the hypothalamus, especially the region of the medial forebrain bundle, is a powerful rewarding area for electrical self-stimulation. The posterior area is a negative rewarding area; stimulation here leading to attack/defence reactions. In the ventromedial nucleus animals will press the lever to receive very short stimuli but longer ones lead to rage (Olds and Olds, 1963). These authors state that stimulation of the human hypothalamus leads to 'euphoria' whereas such stimulation of septal areas leads to a feeling of well-being. Endröczi and Lissák (1962) report that stimulation of the lateral hypothalamus depresses spontaneous motor activity and at higher voltages gives the rage reaction but they claim that it does not interfere with CRs even during the height of the rage reaction. Stimulation of the posterior part of the tuber cinereum, however, gave inhibition of spontaneous activity and of CRs together with vegetative signs of a parasympathetic nature. Lesions in this region that are alleged to improve CAR learning may do so by blocking ACTH release and so decreasing 'anxiety'. Stimulation of the posterior hypothalamus led to increased motor activity and at higher voltages to emotional reactions and a complete suppression of CRs. Stimulation of the lateral hypothalamus can lead to hyper-sexual behaviour.

There is an apparent difference between the effects of HC and hypothalamic stimulation. If the stimulation is introduced once the animal has learned the task, in the case of the HC the animal continues to respond correctly, whereas in the case of the hypothalamus it becomes quite 'confused' again. But this 'confusion' can be overcome if the task concerned is pressing the right lever to deliver an electrical shock to the hypothalamic positive reward area. Thus, in many cases, the suppression of CRs following on hypothalamic stimulation seems to be clearly due to contaminating emotional factors, but this of course may not always necessarily be the case. However, it seems clear that the hypothalamus is prominently concerned with emotional reactions and behaviour of various kinds as well as its vegetative functions.

MacDonnell and Flynn (1966) have demonstrated that the hypothalamus can exert a very specific control of the sensory input different from the more familiar inhibitory mechanisms of selective perception mediated by the RF. In an ordinary cat touching the lips does not evoke any marked response. If however this S is repeated during hypothalamic stimulation, a rapid jaw opening response ensues. The extent of the sensory field from which this response can be evoked is a function of the intensity of the central stimulation. Touching the muzzle during hypothalamic stimulation leads to a head orienting response. Likewise sectioning the sensory nerves to the lips (V) results in the abolition of the jaw opening component of the attack behaviour elicited by stimulation of the hypothalamus. The hypothalamus can thus control specific sequences of S–R that make up the elements of organized patterns of behaviour.

The preoptic area is concerned with temperature regulation. Chronic lesions here lead to a permanently raised heat dissipation threshold and impaired tolerance to cold as well as complete adipsia. Acute lesions are rapidly fatal with hyperpyrexia, hyperglycaemia and a strong sympathetic discharge (Anderson et al, 1965).

The implantation of various steroid hormones into the supraoptic nucleus and anterior medullary eminence leads to increased corticosteroid secretion and altered behaviour. Oestrogen and progesterone implanted in the preoptic area of castrated rats give rise to female mating behaviour. Testosterone, however, did not give rise to male behaviour under these conditions.

Feldman (1962) has made some interesting suggestions concerning hypothalamic function, which will be considered in detail in section 4.3. In brief he supposes that the hypothalamus may bear the same kind of relationship to the allocortex (HC) and the visceral afferents as the thalamus does to neocortex and somatic afferents. It may act also as a way-station on RF–HC control pathways.

3.6 The role of the limbic midbrain area

The RF is well known for its function of alerting the neocortex and its role in sleep and wakefulness. However, it has other important functions besides keeping the cortex awake and it is intimately concerned in learning, conditioned reflexes and limbic activities in general. The limbic midbrain area has massive two-way connections with the HC, septal areas, hypothalamus and amygdala as well as the rest of the RF. Figure 19 gives a general picture of the RF and its connections with the limbic system.

Stimulation of the RF causes widespread neocortical EEG desynchronization and it also has a caudally directed influence affecting transmission through primary sensory relay centres in cord and hindbrain; it also affects muscle tone and posture; and it affects thalamic transmission and controls HC electrical activity. Stimulation of the RF induces HC theta rhythm (probably indicating inhibition of the HC) via the septum–fornix pathway, and the HC in turn probably exercises important inhibitory control over aspects of RF activity.

The RF has an important role in learning and memory. Recent memory is disrupted by RF stimulation. For example, if a rat receives an electric shock at its food cup and the RF is then immediately stimulated it forgets the shock and returns immediately to the cup. Here presumably emotional contamination is not involved. Recent memory in the maze situation is similarly disrupted. Stimulation of the RF abolishes a CR during the period of stimulation and after-discharge (Gastaut, 1958). However, it can also facilitate a CR, or even facilitate one CR and inhibit an antagonistic one at the same time. Stimulation of the neocortex in contradistinction had no effect unless subcortical structures were secondarily involved. On the other hand RF stimulation has been reported not to interfere with new learning in a task where the animal had to learn anew each day which of two levers to press to receive food (Olds and Olds, 1961). Individual neurones in the RF can be conditioned after only 10 pairings of the CS–UCS (Burešová and Bureš, 1965). Stimulation of the dorsomedial tegmentum leads to escape behaviour and hissing and growling responses (MacLean, 1955). Other workers report that RF stimulation gives reactions along the sequence curiosity–attention–(including the orientation response)–fear–terror, together with activation of the pituitary adrenal-stress mechanism according to the stimulus strength used. In unrestrained cats in a social situation RF stimulation leads to quiet behaviour and loss of authority. In monkeys it has been reported to lead to petit-mal-like attacks. Lesions of the ventral central grey in the midbrain abolish a learned response of pressing a lever to avoid a loud noise. There was only a small loss of auditory discriminatory capacity. The lesion seemed to have specifically affected the adverse quality of the painfully loud S (Lyon, 1964). Schiff (1967) has reported that ventral (but not dorsal) tegmental lesions greatly depress the following reactions: bar pressing for septal Ss, saccharin preference thresholds and responsiveness to dim light reward. Thus he concludes that the ventral tegmentum appears to be concerned in reinforcement mechanisms. Thus it would appear that reinforcement depends on an extensive circuit including the HC, amygdala, hypothalamus and the tegmental region. Further details of the role of the RF in learning will be given in chapter 5.

The effect of lesions of the RF are hard to evaluate as, if they are extensive, coma tends to result and partial lesions on so plastic a structure may have no effect. Indeed multiple small lesions have been claimed to have no effect on the CAR nor on the searching response. Unilateral coagulation has been reported, however, to abolish the growling and hissing response derived from stimulation of the ipsilateral amygdala. Sprague and his co-workers (Sprague et al, 1963) suggest on the basis of their lesion experiments cutting the specific lemniscal pathways in the midbrain, that many of the symptoms induced by lesions of the 'RF'—such as defects in attention, orientation, emotional behaviour, and localization—are really due to lesions of the nearby lemniscal pathways.

3.7 The role of various thalamic nuclei

3.7.1 INTRALAMINAR (NON-SPECIFIC) NUCLEI (ILTN)

These nuclei represent the thalamic portion of the reticular formation and appear to be concerned with selective attention in conjunction with areas of neocortex and limbic system. They consist of two main divisions—the reticular nucleus which has many direct cortical connections, and the small midline nuclei which do not. In electrophysiology they are responsible for the well-known recruiting response. Lesions of these nuclei abolish the 'searching response' described above and profoundly disrupt the performance of CRs but they do not affect the spontaneous UCR nor the emotional components of the CR (Thompson, 1963; Knott et al, 1960). Stimulation during a learning response disrupts it.

Kopa et al (1962) have reported some interesting results that throw some light on the extremely important role that these nuclei play in directing behaviour. They trained the animals in a CAR. If the nucleus centrum medianum was stimulated while the animal was on a grid expecting a shock, this resulting in increased fear, restlessness, and it activated the pre-established CAR. If, however, this nucleus was stimulated while the animal was on the bench where it had never been shocked, general relaxation resulted and the cat took up its usual sleeping posture.

Stimuli here can activate a previously established CR. If an animal has learned two CRs, one a CAR and one an alimentary one, the stimulation will activate both if the animal is hungry but only the former if it is not. Thus stimulation of this nucleus will activate a CR only if the relevant drive is present (e.g. fear or hunger as the case may be). Stimulation can also lead to activation of the pituitary/adrenal axis and lesions to abolition of the HC theta rhythm. Atropine injected into the reticular thalamic nucleus impaired both appetitive (black–white discrimination) and aversive training: applied to the midline nuclei it had the opposite effect. Simple sensorimotor functions were unaffected (Grossman and Peters, 1966). Carbachol injections in the reticular nucleus also greatly impaired the acquisition of aversive and alimentary conditioned reflexes, but had no effect on exploratory behaviour or on food or water intake. In the midline thalamic nuclei, on the other hand, it depressed exploratory behaviour and delayed CAR learning (Grossman et al, 1965). Therefore, they supposed that the reticular nuclei may be concerned with the acquisition, retention and recall of conditioned reflexes and the midline nuclei may be related to non-specific motivational processes (e.g. attention, activation). Bohus and de Wied (1967) however, on the basis of lesion experiments, came to a different conclusion, namely that the small midline nuclei may be concerned with the acquisition of conditioned reflexes and the nucleus parafascicularis with motivational factors.

Thus these nuclei clearly play an important part in attention, conditioned reflexes and learning. This will be described in more detail in chapter 5.

3.7.2 THE DORSOMEDIAL NUCLEUS

This has close anatomical connections with the hypothalamus and the orbitofrontal neocortex. It is familiar to psychiatrists as the target nucleus in the operation of thalamotomy, where the nucleus itself is coagulated and in prefrontal leucotomy where its connections to the orbitofrontal cortex are severed. These operations appear to reduce emotional 'tension', 'anxiety' and 'agitation'. Using Olds's technique this nucleus can be shown to be a negative rewarding area, and stimulation here is punishing, according to Olds, leading to fear and escape reactions and the animal will press the lever to switch off the stimulating current.* Destruction

---

* Some experiments by Valenstein and Valenstein (1964) have, however, cast doubt on the supposition that we can deduce that an S is adversive just because the animal switches it off. They find that animals will repetitively turn on and off electrical self-stimulation in many areas and, moreover, that, whereas higher intensity of S causes them to switch off sooner, it also causes them to switch on again sooner. They quote Kavanar (1964) as finding that animals will repeatedly switch on and off any S under their control. The authors raise '. . . a critical question about the nature of the presumed aversion which results from prolonged positive stimulation'. This criticism refers, however, to the situation described, in which the fact that the animals switched off after a reasonable period of switching on led to the hypothesis that an originally rewarding S had turned negative (by some mechanism such as recruitment of

of this nucleus leads to decreased escape behaviour. There seemed to be no loss of fear drive and, in animals at any rate, this nucleus was thought to operate on the higher control of the motor response to fear rather than on the fear drive itself (Roberts and Carey, 1963). Thompson (1963) has reported that lesions here disrupt CARs to visual but not to auditory stimuli and (Knott et al, 1960) that they disrupt the lever pressing response for food. Olton and Isaacson (1967) found that lesions of the nucleus had no effect on fear motivation as measured by extinction rates of an active avoidance response, but they reduced re-acquisition rates. They suggest that the nucleus functions in this task by mediating 'fear' as a function of the immediate stimulus and that it does not mediate 'fear' in response to some internal representation of the S, or in response to other S associated with the original S by stimulus generalization. This may of course reflect contaminating emotional factors or non-specific unresponsiveness rather than interference with specific learning mechanisms. Stimulation of this nucleus in an unrestrained monkey gave a reliable sequence of somewhat meaningless behaviour—walking to the cage wall, jumping up and hanging on for a while and then walking back to the starting point.

3.7.3 ANTERIOR NUCLEI

These lie on the HC–cingulate pathway (both direct and via the mamillary bodies). Lesions here induce altered states of consciousness and a marked reduction in the emotional response of cats to noxious stimuli (Baird et al, 1951). Stimulation can lead to an alerting response or to confusion.

3.8 Miscellaneous regions

3.8.1 THE EXTRAPYRAMIDAL BASAL GANGLIA

The HC and entorhinal area do not appear to connect directly to the basal ganglia but the amygdala does. Connections also run from the ILTN to the head of the caudate nucleus and the putamen, and the sleeping cat can be awakened by electrical stimula-

---

effects in the subliminal fringe). It may not apply to cases where the animal rapidly switches off the current that the experimenter has switched on.

tion of the amygdala and globus pallidus in a manner similar to RF stimulation. There is a variety of somewhat disconnected reports in the literature. Lesions of the putamen and dorsal globus pallidus have no apparent effect on the CAR in the monkey. Lesions of the globus pallidus have been reported to depress retention of a kinaesthetic habit in rats. However, lesions in this region can lead to hypokinetic reactions (Carey, 1957), which may contaminate the results. Stimulation of the caudate nucleus depresses the ability of the monkey to execute a delayed alternation task. Caudate lesions affect the localization of auditory clues and the ability to find one's way around in familiar surroundings. Lesions in the globus pallidus in cats tested for CAR, increased the rate of extinction of the reaction markedly and increased the reaction time (Laursen, 1962). Similar lesions in the nucleus centrum medianum of the thalamus had no such effect and indeed decreased the RT. The parameters of the electrical stimulus used have in this case as in others been shown to be of vital importance. Caudate stimulation at low frequency (5 c/s) induces sleep, at high frequency (35–90 c/s) arousal, and at intermediate frequencies (20–30 c/s) an arrest-like reaction. Parts of the caudate nucleus induce reactions similar to those induced from the nearby septum, e.g. motor inhibition and loss of interest for food. Evidence that the globus pallidus may be concerned in timing behaviour is presented by Brady and Conrad (1960). These interesting experiments need further development before any firm interpretations can be made.

Travis et al (1968) made unit recordings from the globus pallidus in monkeys during food-motivated behaviour. Many units were inhibited only during particular sequences of food-motivated behaviour (e.g. searching for food pellet, carrying pellet to mouth, etc.). The same movements with inedible objects resulted in no such inhibition. The authors see behaviour as compound of a chain of S–R units, for example

S_1	→	R_1	→	S_2	→	R_2	→	S_3	→	R_3	→	S_4	→	R_4
lever		press		food		search		food in		carry		food in		EAT
out		lever		hopper		for food		hand		food to		mouth		
										mouth				

G

In these experiments each S–R situation was associated with the inhibition of a different pattern of pallidal neurones. The initiation of the inhibition was conditional on highly specific sensory inputs which immediately guide behaviour by reinforcement. They conclude that '. . . the globus pallidus is in a position to interrelate cortical and subcortical mechanisms of movement with diencephalic motivational mechanisms and to give neurophysiological priority to specific stimulus–response sequences involved in food related behaviour'.

3.8.2. THE SUBTHALAMIC AREA

This region is located astride the important direct HC–RF pathways and Adey et al (1962) have recently studied the effect of lesions here. In cats recording electrodes were placed in the HC, subthalamus and midbrain limbic area. Unilateral coagulation of the subthalamus led to the following behavioural effects: (1) great distractibility during a forced delayed response period (e.g. when food is placed under one of a number of cups but the animal is restrained from approaching for some time) (2) animals failed to approach food hidden under a cup in the opposite visual field even though they had carefully watched it put there (3) the slow wave frequency during the approach in the HC dropped from 6 c/s to 4 c/s and the concurrent slow waves in the RF and sensorimotor cortex (that normally run at the same frequency as the HC slow waves) became quite irregular. Bilateral lesions led to gross impairment of delayed reactions. As soon as the food was concealed the cat's attention wandered. The EEG rhythms in the HC were still further disrupted and the RF and sensorimotor cortex became devoid of electrical activity.

These lesions probably operate by reason of the disruption of the HC–RF pathways. The results indicate the importance of the flow of information about the environment processed by the HC (and it appears specifically ipsilaterally at this stage) and the effect of this on attention and recent memory; as well as the interdependence between the HC, diencephalon and neocortex in the maintenance of their normal EEG rhythms. Removal of the entorhinal area is associated with the development of sleep spindles in the auditory cortex. Therefore the entorhinal area must affect diencephalocortical relations. No other cortical region produces this result. Tonic influences from the sub-thalamus are necessary for maintaining the responsiveness of the RF (Lindsley et al, 1968). Lesions here reduced the evoked potentials in the RF following sensory stimulation and affects the excitability of RF neurones. The afferent inflow to the sub-thalamus comes widely from limbic and neocortical areas.

3.9 The role of neocortex and juxtallocortex

The major components of the limbic system—the hippocampus and the amygdala—are closely related to the neocortex of the medial aspect of the cerebral hemispheres, in particular to the orbitofrontal region and much of the temporal lobe neocortex. The transitional band of cortex between the ancient allocortex and the more recently developed neocortex is called juxtallocortex. Its major divisions are the cingulate cortex (also called 'mesocortex'), the presubiculum and parts of the orbito-insular-temporal cortex ('frontotemporal' cortex).

3.9.1 THE TEMPORAL LOBE

Much of the information that we possess on the limbic functions of the cortex has come from Penfield and his co-workers in their studies on temporal lobe epilepsy and the effect of stimulating the cortex in conscious subjects. Penfield's work suggests that temporal lobe cortex seems to be concerned with the interpretation of experience, with certain complex sensory functions and possibly with laying down of permanent memory stores. It shares various visceral functions common to 'frontotemporal' cortex. The superior and lateral portions of the temporal lobe seem to be concerned with sensory function. Stimulation here in conscious subjects leads to *interpretative illusions*:

(*a*) sounds seem louder or fainter, nearer or further, clearer or less distinct;

(*b*) visual objects look larger or smaller, nearer or further, clearer or blurred, and their apparent speed of movement may be altered;

(c) recognition is affected in that present experience may be endowed with a feeling of illusory familiarity (*deja vu*) or alternatively a familiar scene may appear unfamiliar, strange, unreal, wierd or altered in some undefinable way;

(d) also to various emotions such as fear, loneliness, sorrow or disgust.

Presumably these findings indicate that the temporal cortex acts as a sort of fine control over various aspects of vision and audition as well as inducing certain emotional reactions including the most interesting 'feeling' of familiarity or strangeness that so links perception, emotion and memory. The temporal cortex also seems to act as a sort of detailed memory store in which a continuous record of our experiences can be stored complete with the emotions felt at that time. Stimulation here can release these past experiences in a particularly vivid form which feels to the subject as if he were actually reliving the events recalled. Penfield supposes on a basis of this well-known evidence that 'the temporal cortex compares present and past experiences . . . whether this has been experienced before, wherein strange, wherein familiar, whether fearful . . .' He suggests that this record is stored as a record of continued experience, as on a video-tape recorder, as well as in a classified form, e.g. all 'snatching experiences', all sounds, or sight, with certain common qualities ('red', 'square', 'happened on Thursday', etc.).

The criticism has been made that these changes have only been found in epileptic subjects and in only a few of these. The possibility remains, therefore, that some of these findings represent pathological function in epilepsy. However, it seems more plausible that the epileptic lesion merely renders the physiological function of the cortex amenable to release by the unphysiological stimuli used. It seems rather improbable that an epileptic lesion could induce *de novo* such complex functions in a cortex whose real function was something quite different. However, it is possible that the record of these experiences with their concomitant emotions, or the classified type of memory described above, the actual evaluation of the familiarity or otherwise of the sensory information, its analysis in terms of classified categories and the linking of sensory information with appropriate emotions and behaviour may all be done in the various limbic circuits (as suggested more fully in chapter 6) in which the temporal lobe cortex may have an essential function. Adey (1965) states: '. . . I am inclined to think that the notion of interdependence between temporal lobe structures and the diencephalon are the critical determinants of eliciting these stored images.' Sem-Jacobsen and Torkildsen (1960) report two types of memory recall following stimulation of the temporal lobe: (1) a precise type (like video-tape) elicited from the medial side close to the HC and (2) confused hallucinatory fragments from more posterior regions close to the parietal lobe. Penfield had described on the other hand a rather sudden transition from mere flashes of light and formless hallucinations provoked by stimulating visual cortex to fully formed memories from temporal cortex. These workers also report various types of emotional responses which they described as either 'positive' (a feeling of ease and relaxation with joy and smiling) or 'negative' (restlessness, depression, fright, horror). However, the interpretation as to what emotion was actually concerned was not always simple. One case responding with laughter said afterwards she laughed because she was really being 'tickled'. The positive and negative areas were often quite close together. Mild to moderate effects were obtained from the temporal lobe and the ventromedial part of the frontal lobe. In the frontal lobe the 'relaxing' area was ventromedial to the 'anxiety' area. Strong emotional reactions were obtained from midline regions around the third ventricle and from the mesencephalon. They noted little effect from unilateral stimulation of the HC. Stimulation of points in the anterior temporal, cingulate and orbitofrontal gyri led to the autonomic changes to be described in detail in the next section.

In monkeys ablation of temporal lobe cortex impairs visual discrimination (for both new and old learning). This learning appears to be conducted by corticocortical pathways from the parastriate to temporal regions since it was unaffected by cutting thalamocortical pathways or by cortical undercutting but is abolished by cortical ablations or cross-hatching (Chow, 1961).

There is some evidence that the left temporal lobe is more concerned with speech (in particular with the understanding and retention of verbally expressed ideas) and the right lobe with rapid visual identification.

3.9.2. THE CINGULATE GYRUS AND ORBITO-TEMPORAL-INSULAR CORTEX

The orbito-temporal-insular cortex consists of the sheet of cortex in the depths of the sylvian fissure that takes in the posterior part of the orbital surface of the frontal lobe, the medial part of the temporal lobe, much of the insula and connecting bits of cortex in between these. It consists of juxtallocortex and has much in common functionally with the cingulate gyrus—so much so that they can be considered together.

3.9.2 *a*. STIMULATION EXPERIMENTS
Somatomotor effects

Respiratory movements. Stimulation of the cingulate gyrus leads to an arrest of respiration in expiration. This seems to be part of a more generalized inhibition of motor activity. The inhibition lasts for a variable length of time, depending on the species, then respiratory escape occurs. In man one gets the same effect associated with feelings of sleepiness, tiredness and impaired consciousness. This effect is also obtained from much of the rest of the orbito-temporal-insular cortex (OTIC). In some instances acceleration of respiratory movements has been reported—from middle and anterior cingulate cortex (dog)—where it may represent the common dual representation of opposite functions for control of a single system in closely adjacent areas of the limbic system (cf. the amygdala). This arrangement would seem to offer advantages for a system concerned with homeostatic control. Acceleration of respiration has also been reported from stimulating the peri-amygdaloid cortex where it may represent a different function—e.g. sniffing associated with the known olfactory functions of this part of the brain.

Inhibition of motor movement and tone. Stimulation of the anterior cingulate region gives inhibition of all spontaneous movement, a decrease in muscle tone and sleep. In other regions of OTIC one gets an arrest of spontaneous movement without an effect on tone. Such stimulation can also lead to modulation of movements induced by stimulation of the motor cortex; these may be inhibited, augmented or first one and then the other. This area can be regarded in part as a sensorimotor vagal area and many of the effects of stimulating it can be obtained by stimulating the central cut end of the vagus. An anatomical pathway has been demonstrated running from the vagal nuclei to the anterior cingulate region (via the anterior hypothalamus and the septal area). Presumably there must also be close connections with the sympathetic system. The region may represent an area whereby emotional factors can influence motor movements, tone and behaviour.

Tonic and clonic movements. These movements are obtained in anaesthetized animals and presumably represent fragments of the more complex behaviour sequences seen in unanaesthetized animals. These movements survive bilateral extirpation of the motor cortex, illustrating again the semi-independence of control of 'emotional' movements as opposed to 'voluntary' ones. This is, of course, a fact also commonly seen in clinical experience in cases of brain damage and such conditions as cerebral palsy.

Vocalization, chewing, licking, swallowing. These may all be obtained from the cingulate area. Vocalization may be obtained from monkey and dog (but not as yet cat) from the anterior cingulate and HC gyri in a manner not to suggest a mere reaction to pain.

Autonomic responses

Blood pressure. Stimulation of OTIC reveals interlaced areas for producing depression and elevation of blood pressure.

Gastric motility. There are two areas on the lateral surface of the hemisphere and a small area of the pre- and sub-callosal region that give inhibition of pyloric peristalsis and an increase of intestinal peristalsis. Stimulation of the olfactory bulb also gives a sizeable increase in gastric motility. The latter is, of course, powerfully affected by emotional changes and by olfactory stimuli of suitable gastronomic power.

Pupillary responses. All regions of OTIC that give the arousal response also give rise to pupillary dilatation. This is best seen from the precallosal region. The regions that give the opposite sleep-like responses give rise similarly to pupillary constriction. This is best obtained from the anterior cingulate region near the genu of the corpus callosum.

Miscellaneous reactions. Other vegetative responses that may be obtained include piloerection, salivation, bladder contraction and defaecation. All these autonomic responses mentioned are mediated by pathways running to the brainstem, mainly, it is probable, via the hypothalamic pathway. It is also concerned in the secretion of insulin.

Behaviour

A typical arousal response may be obtained by stimulation of the cingulate cortex and from parts of OTIC as well as from sites in temporal isocortex, frontal eye cortex, sensorimotor cortex and the paraoccipital region. This response is mediated via the intralaminar thalamic nuclei, destruction of which abolishes the response.

Ablation experiments. It is curious that lesions of this region do not lead to any observable effects on the vegetative functions that are affected so powerfully by stimulation of the region. Lesions lead to no effect on motor performance, muscle tone, respiration, cardiovascular or gastrointestinal function, the pupils, etc. The only change reported is a decreased resistance to oxygen lack. Decortication of the basal temporal cortex leads to an increase of the excitability of the amygdala and HC. The main changes from such ablations are behavioural.

Behavioural changes

Lesions of the cingulate gyrus were described by Pechtel et al (1958) to lead to the following results: (*a*) amnesia for previous learning (*b*) impairment of new learning skills (*c*) a tendency to diffuse and precipitate activity and (*d*) increased aggression and a lowered threshold for fear and startle. Previous studies had suggested that cingulate lesions led to increased tameness rather than aggression (monkey, cat) and a reduction of hostility, fear and tension in humans. Immediately following the operation in cats a peculiar but transient change has been reported consisting of confused and perseverative behaviour (the so-called Kennard syndrome—which may be due to damage to the posterior granular cingulate cortex). In humans some disturbance has been reported in the temporal ordering of recent events.

Thomas and Slotnick (1962) suggested that the cingulate region has no basic effect on learning but that it serves to inhibit the 'freezing' element of the CER. Very frightened animals will 'freeze' and this response is clearly incompatible with the CAR where the animal must escape. This conflict does not arise in maze learning (where the animals are not frightened) and this would explain why cingulate lesions affect the CAR but not maze learning. Thomas and Slotnick (1962) report that cingulate lesions in monkeys induce no change in emotionality, social dominance or aggressiveness, nor as we noted in maze learning, but only on the acquisition of the CAR. This hypothesis (that the CAR is impaired because the incompatible 'freezing' element of the CER cannot be inhibited) was tested by comparing the effect of cingulectomy on CAR performance under high as opposed to low hunger drive. High hunger drive inhibits the tendency to 'freeze' and in this experiment the hungry rats with cingulate lesions showed no tendency to 'freeze' and normal CAR performance. This supports the author's claim that the cingular gyrus has no direct concern with memory or learning but rather with emotional responses, and particularly perhaps with the motor aspects of emotional responses, disorders of which can secondarily interfere with learning and memory—as we have seen to be the case in other parts of the limbic system. Peretz (1960) has produced some supportive evidence in that cingulectomy in rats depressed the CAR but improved visual discrimination performance and increased the bar-pressing rate under hunger drive.

Thomas and Otis (1958a) produced similar excessive 'freezing' by lesions of the projection fibres from the anterior thalamic nucleus to the cingulate gyrus, without any gross change in emotionality. Their lesions also included the rostral HC, however, and this might explain why their animals also showed impaired maze learning (Thomas and Otis, 1958b). This effect of producing excessive 'freezing' was traced still further back along the Papez circuit by Thomas et al (1963) who produced it by making lesions in the mamillothalamic tract. This produced marked apparent disturbances in the retention and relearning of CARs but no interference with a positively reinforced visual discrimination response. They concluded that these results were due to the release of the innate defensive reaction of 'freezing' without any effect on recent memory.

A contrary view is entered by Kimble and Gostnell (1968). They were able to demonstrate a severe deficit in the acquisition of a CAR (two-way shuttle box) in cingulate rats, but failed to find any significant differences in two separate measures of 'emotionality'. Their controls were rats with neocortical and HC lesions. They felt that these results gave no support for the 'increased freezing response' hypothesis but supported instead the Barker–Thomas hypothesis which suggests that the cingulate gyrus is concerned with organizing temporal sequences of behaviour. Barker (1967) tested the retention of sequence-learning following cingulate lesions. He found that lesions in the anterior cingulate region markedly impaired performance of 2- and 4-lever sequences, increasing both sequential and perseverative errors. Lesions in the posterior region or in the neocortex had no effect. The most convincing evidence comes from some studies carried out by Slotnick (1967), who studied the effects of cingulate lesions on maternal behaviour. All the motor patterns seen in normal rats were seen but they were carried out in an irregular and confused manner. Pups were repeatedly brought in and out of the cage and dropped randomly about. The mothers showed little inclination to nurse the pups; they might adopt the nursing position over one or two pups but the rest were ignored, and the mothers spent much of their time sniffing about the cage. The behaviour improved and became almost normal by the 4th day, but it could be easily disrupted by making small changes in the environment. The behavioural defect correlated with the degree of severity of retrograde degeneration in the anterior thalamic nuclei. Slotnick concludes that the cingulate cortex participates in the control of complex unlearned sequences of behaviour. The defect in maternal care was not due to indifference but to inappropriate, though well-motivated, responses to pups and nesting material.

Chapter 4

SOME ASPECTS OF

THE ELECTRICAL ACTIVITY

OF LIMBIC AREAS

This section will deal with certain aspects of the electrical activity of the limbic system, in particular with the HC theta rhythm, the fast rhythm of the amygdala, some RF–hypothalamus–HC relationships and seizure activity. Other aspects will be dealt with in chapter 5 where these impinge on learning and CR formation.

4.1 The hippocampal theta rhythm

During depth recordings from unanaesthetized animals a prominent theta rhythm of around 5–7 c/s can be recorded from the HC. This rhythm is characteristic of the carnivores and lagomorphs. 'It is much more difficult to discern in the monkey, and our data from the chimpanzee indicate a complex form of rhythmic activity that is usually well above the theta band in frequency. Human hippocampal records also show a great deal of faster activity than that to be found in the theta band' (Adey, 1965). As we noted above the theta rhythm is evoked by RF activation via a pathway running through the hypothalamus, septum and fornix. The septal cells fire in synchrony with theta. It is also dependent on the centromedian nucleus of the thalamus. It is not affected on destruction of the entorhinal area. This rhythm was at first regarded as the arousal response of the HC as it seemed to be evoked by a new stimulus. It thus appeared that the arousal pattern of archicortex was represented by a hypersynchronous burst of theta rhythm in contradistinction to the desynchronization that marks neocortical arousal. However, it has since been suggested that the first response of the HC to a completely novel stimulus is desynchronization. In this view, the 5–7 c/s pattern is probably really a sign of inhibition of the HC. During conditioning the time course of the HC theta rhythm is the same as the time course of the orienting response. The latter response in turn is replaced by the stabilized conditioned reflex. When this occurs the theta rhythm dies away, the HC is again activated and this inhibits the RF thus cutting short the orienting response (for which the RF is responsible) and so allowing the fully developed CR to materialize. The HC certainly can inhibit the RF; the RF controls the orienting response and this must be inhibited before the animal can go, e.g. to the food tray to complete the CR. This view therefore is that the theta rhythm is merely a sign of relative HC inactivity.

The HC theta rhythm is seen only if the S is familiar in some respect. The normal response to a totally new S is a startle reaction with HC fast activity. Pickenhain and Klingberg (1967) characterize the behavioural reaction in which HC theta appears as '... one in which the animal compares the actual sensory information coming from the situation with previously stored information'. In a shock avoidance test, if the CS is ten consecutive light-flashes, a well trained rat will make an avoidance reaction on the seventh or eighth flash. At the first flash no HC reaction occurs. Then theta builds up and reaches a maximum just before the rat jumps to safety. With positive reinforcement conditioning, HC theta is prominent during training but once the rat is fully conditioned, it goes. Thus HC theta 'appears in all behavioural situations in which the rat displays a motivated behaviour'. The frequency of the rhythm is a direct function of the degree of motivation.

Adey (1967), correlates the HC theta rhythm with approach behaviour, with the execution of a planned motor act and with imprinting information of importance during the learning process. It seems possible, however, that the rhythm may subserve *more than one* function, i.e. it may signify inhibition of the HC–RF control by inhibition of axonal efferent activity by reason of excessive slow wave activity in dendrites; this latter may also however favour some manner of imprinting of important information or mediating patterns of motivation and/or executive control of behaviour. These aspects will be discussed in more detail in chapter 5.

Adey (1965) wrote as follows:

'There is not the slightest doubt that hippocampal theta activity in the range from 4 to 7 cycles per second is continuously present in the alerted animal and that in the presence of a completely novel stimulus it merely synchronizes to a more regular character. The critical parameter appears to be location of the electrodes within the hippocampus. In the paper by Porter *et al* (1964) we used an array of electrodes less than 2 millimeters apart spanning the hippocampus, both longitudinally and transversely. By this technique we are able for the first time to discern the fine regional differences in the chronic animal. It was apparent that the region of the hippocampal pyramidal dendritic layer is associated with continuous theta activity. By contrast, more ventral regions around the dentate fascia, and in the vicinity of the subiculum, frequently showed essentially desynchronized records until either orienting behaviour or a discrimination was required. In these circumstances both types of record took on a rhythmicity at around 6 cycles per second during the discriminative performance. Nor is the theta rhythm associated specifically with orienting behaviour. By computer analysis, we have confirmed the presence of the 6 cycle per second activity as a concomitant of discriminative behaviour, and a 4 cycle rhythmicity as characteristic of orientation. Moreover, by the use of psychotomimetic agents, such as LSD and the cyclohexamines, we have achieved a lasting separation of the two types of behaviour and the concomitant rhythmic processes.'

Adey suggests that an individual neurone may be viewed as a phase comparator of electronic processes sweeping across its dendritic surface in complex spatio-temporal patterns. The excitability of a cortical neurone may depend on the relationship of the wave pattern at the cell surface to an 'optimal' pattern of waves determined by the previous history of the cell in a stochastic probabilistic mode of operation.

Petsche and Stumpf (1960), however, used a multi-electrode toposcopic response to examine this apparent phase shift and were inclined to attribute it instead to differences of frequency and rate of propagation which appeared to depend on the location of the recording electrode on various parts of the HC. However, the experimental situations may not have been strictly comparable.

Power spectrum analysis (Elazar and Adey, 1967) has defined more closely the shifts in the frequency of HC theta during different stages of the performance of a well-learned response. An alert animal in the pre-S stage shows a wide variety of theta (3–7 c/s) with a peak at 4 c/s. The stimulus shifts this peak to 5 c/s, the approach period shifts it to 6 c/s and after performance of the task, it drops back to 4 c/s. If an incorrect response is made the 6 c/s peak is missing from the record taken during the approach period and in fact the 6 c/s rhythm was never seen except during successful approach behaviour. These rhythms and peaks appear also in other areas (e.g. amygdala, subthalamus, RF and cortex) with subtle modifications and there is a high degree of linear correlation between rhythms in these various areas. The HC waves are organized in a very regular and consistent manner but in the other structures they are much more irregular and variable. The authors see the HC as taking a leading role in complex interacting neuronal circuits activated during the consolidation of learning.

This concept of the function of the HC theta rhythm is supported by Vanderwolf and Heron (1964) who made recordings from the medial hypothalamus of the rat during the performance of a CAR in a two-way shuttle box. A train of regular 6–9 c/s waves often appeared 1–5 seconds before the response was made. These were seldom seen in the hypothalamus at other times. They were very similar in appearance to HC theta and appeared to be related to planned action.

Brown (1968) measured the HC theta during various behavioural responses in the cat. The rhythm became more regular as a function of the degree of attention, particularly visual attention, and there was no necessary connection with movement. The HC theta was felt to be related to the discrimination of the significance of the sensory S. Phase shifts appeared to be a function of frequency changes and did not seem to have any special relation to stages in the learning process.

Further support for Adey's ideas (i.e. that the HC theta is related to goal-directed behaviour as against Grastyán's theory—that it is concerned with the orienting reflex—is reported by Bremner (1964). In HC recordings taken during the performance of a Sidman avoidance schedule, the HC becomes very regular (at 5–7 c/s) just before and during the lever press. Electrical stimulation of the HC at 3 c/s drove the HC EEG at this frequency until just before the lever press when the theta rhythm broke through.

In a recent paper Grastyán et al (1966) postulate the existence of two basic mechanisms in the brain: 'approach' and 'run away' mechanisms. They stimulated the hypothalamus in the cat and recorded from the HC. Low-voltage stimuli gave an orienting reaction, HC theta was evoked and the animal walked about. If it pressed the lever that switched off the S, there was an immediate adversive reaction to the pedal together with desynchronization of the HC rhythm. Repeated S now led to a conditioned avoidance of the pedal. High-voltage stimuli in exactly the same place led to an immediate HC desynchronization and flight. If the lever was now pressed, the S was again switched off and this led to an immediate return of the HC theta. Repeating the S now led to a conditioned approach reaction to the pedal. Other hypothalamic loci were found that gave one or other of these effects but not both (lateral—'approach'; medial and posterior—'avoid'). They therefore distinguished successive phases in the formation of a conditioned reflex. (1) The stage of diffuse orientation, or orientation directed at the source of the S—not the goal—marked by HC theta getting faster. (2) The stage of goal-directed behaviour, marked by HC desynchronization. A train of theta waves follows the completion of the motor consummatory act. The results were the same for both approach and avoidance behaviour. They then conditioned an approach and an avoidance reaction in the same animal to sounds of different pitch. Avoidance of both reactions was obtained by low-voltage S of the hypothalamus which induced HC theta. Activation of the conditioned reflex was achieved only by higher voltage S, strong enough to cause HC desynchronization. The threshold voltage required to activate the avoidance reaction was always lower than that required to activate the approach reaction. The theta rhythm returned once the food had been eaten or the animal was relaxed in a safe place.

The authors interpret their results as indicating that the HC controls a homeostatic mechanism in which action builds up counter-action by a process of negative feedback. A moderate 'motivational state' induced by mild stimulation of the hypothalamus evokes HC theta and release of the approach function, whereas a stronger 'motivational state' induced by stronger stimulation gives HC fast activity and release of the avoidance reaction. If the animal attends to a series of stimuli, this naturally results in a sequence of (pull–push) reactions as attention to one object must be inhibited before attention to the next object can occur. Thus in Grastyán's view the HC theta mediates a non-specific motivational process and he raises the interesting question of the possible role of the rebound phenomena once the S has been switched off. On the other hand HC theta may signal 'reinforcement possible' or 'reinforcement received', whereas HC desynchronization may be a concomitant of putting into action sequences of motor behaviour required to achieve reinforcement whether this is food or the cessation of pain. Thus it is clear that there is still considerable disagreement of the facts concerning HC theta, let alone its interpretation.

If records are taken from the HC during electrical self-stimulation the HC usually shows fast waves (30–40 c/s), sometimes desynchronization and never theta. Conversely stimulation of points which produce HC theta never produces self-stimulation.

The fact that the HC modulates lower autonomic and motor structures has not been the focus of as much research as has been directed towards its participation in 'higher' mental functions (motivation, learning, etc.). Yokata and Fujimori (1964) showed that HC synchronization, produced by stimulation of the medial preoptic area, medial hypothalamus or dorsal tegmentum, was

H

associated with the facilitation of monosynaptic reflexes in the spinal cord, a rise in BP and changes in skin potentials. HC desynchronization, produced by stimulation of the lateral preoptic area or amygdala, was associated with a lower BP and inhibition of the cord reflexes. Likewise an upward spread of HC theta was reported by Yamaguchi et al (1967). They described an 'isohippocampal rhythm' (IHR) which is a theta rhythm in the cortex waxing and waning in conjunction with the HC theta. It is prominent in occipital and temporal areas. It augments and regularizes the primary cortical potentials evoked in the cortex by stimulation of the lateral or medial geniculate. The IHR appears in some cortical areas just before the performance of a lever press for food reward, also just before the performance of a defensive conditioned reflex. Radulovacki and Adey (1965) suggest that the complex rhythms of the HC are transmitted elsewhere and may subserve memory function. Memory recall may depend on the stochastic re-establishment of similar wave patterns. The HC theta also appears to be related to some HC action that synchronizes the activity of various thalamic nuclei (Manzoni and Parmeggiani, 1964) and in wider brain areas including cortex (Manzoni and Parmeggiani, 1965).

Stimulation of the vagus can induce two reactions depending on the type of fibre stimulated. High frequency, low voltage S gives cortical and thalamic synchronization and disrupts HC theta. All other S give cortical and thalamic desynchronization and marked HC theta (Chase et al, 1966).

The HC theta rhythm is very prominent during sleep when the cortex sustains an alert pattern. If the HC is stimulated during this phase the sleep changes over to the slow wave type. Lesse et al (1955) report that a characteristic 14–17 c/s rhythm occurs in human HC during recollections of past events of special emotional significance. These were never seen during the mere expression of emotion without specific recollection. It did not spread to other subcortical or cortical regions. Guerrero-Figueroa and Heath (1964) have recorded the potentials evoked in the HC by stimulation of the centromedian nucleus of the thalamus in man. Under relaxed conditions this has the form of a rapid initial component (a di- or tri-phasic complex) of short latency followed by a large slow wave response and then a second complex rather similar to the first some 300–500 m.sec later. When the subject did mental arithmetic or showed an emotional reaction the form of the initial component was unchanged but this was now followed by a train of smaller and more regular waves.

It is generally agreed that evoked responses in the HC are complex and labile and are easily modified by slight changes in position of these recording or stimulating electrodes (Green, 1964). An 'inactivation process' has been described for the HC: this is a series of waves close to the theta rhythm in frequency caused by a burst of firing of HC cells above a certain critical frequency. A phase of hyperpolarization follows an initial phase of depolarization, and successive potentials of the firing cells are progressively attenuated. This may represent a defence against the explosive tendency of the HC to seizure activity. The 'inactivation process' is triggered by the same stimuli that trigger the theta rhythm and is likewise blocked by septal faradization.

The HC record from humans is rather a colourless affair compared with the rabbit. Pagni and Marossero (1965) report that there is nothing specific about the resting rhythm and that there is no arousal response and no theta rhythm.

Physostigmine induces, and atropine reduces, HC theta, suggesting a cholinergic mechanism. LSD also inhibits HC theta as an immediate response and this is followed for 3 days by an increase in the amplitude and regularity of the rhythm (Adey, 1967).

4.2 The amygdala fast rhythm

The basolateral amygdala also has a characteristic rhythm of about 40–45 c/s (Lesse, 1960). This is evoked by a meaningful or noxious stimulus (food, water, proximity of mouse or dog, loud noises, etc.). It is not seen in the corticomedial division nor in other parts of the limbic system. It does not occur during simple arousal from sleep. It appears before avoidance learning becomes evident and persists long after such learning has been extinguished. Grastyán (1961) has suggested that this rhythm indicates the general level of unconditioned mechanisms and drives. It may also represent an 'alerting' alarm call to the amygdala to operate quickly in conditions where its functions in reinforcement and reaction to meaningful stimuli and its role in alerting the pituitary–adrenal axis may be called for.

Adey (1965) has indicated its essential inflexibility in relation to the actual task performance, '. . . thereby contrasting very sharply with the exquisite plasticity of hippocampal rhythms. We confirmed the decline of the 40 c/s activity in satiation of hunger.' John and Killam (1959) on the other hand, claim that this rhythm appears in cat amygdala during CAR training only when the animal reaches 100 per cent criterion, and in this case usually immediately precedes the performance of the CAR itself.

Wepsic and Sutin (1964) have demonstrated by physiological means an afferent inflow to the central and basal nuclei of the amygdala from the magnocellular part of the medial geniculate body. Stimulation of the latter (and the septum) leads to evoked responses (latency 12–23 m.sec) in the amygdala and also to firing or modulation of single units therein. These single units responded to auditory stimuli and to nasal air puffs but not apparently (in anaesthetized cats, anyway) to tactile, nociceptive and photic stimuli. Single unit analysis showed that septal stimulation and geniculate stimulation activated different neurones. This region of the medial geniculate (the phylogenetically older part) has extensive connections to the secondary sensory areas in the temporal lobe. However, this response is not mediated by this route as it was not abolished by ablation of the temporal neocortex. This route may form part of the 'alert to danger' function of the amygdala as this part of the medial geniculate has been linked to nociceptive stimulation over large areas of body wall: on the other hand, these present experimenters failed to fire amygdala single units by nociceptive stimuli—possibly the anaesthetic used might account for this. The 40 c/s rhythm of the amygdala is conducted into the olfactory bulb. This has a basic faster rhythm which gets overridden. An olfactory S in an alert cat inhibits the 40 c/s rhythm in the amygdala, whereas in an inattentive cat, it potentiates it (McLennan and Greystone, 1965). Thus this rhythm may represent a gated system scanning for an olfactory input.

4.3 Feldman's hypothesis

Feldman (1962) has suggested some interesting analogies between the RF–thalamic–neocortical relationship on the one hand and the RF–hypothalamic–archicortical (HC) relationship on the other. Sciatic nerve stimulation gives rise to long-latency evoked potentials in the anterior and medial hypothalamus, preoptic area and septum (as well as in the RF) and to short-latency evoked potentials in the posterior and lateral hypothalamus (like those seen in the medial lemniscus). Simultaneous stimulation of the RF, HC or amygdala *inhibits* these potentials in hypothalamus, preoptic area and septum. The hypothalamus in turn connects to the HC via many short latency monosynaptic pathways together with some slower polysynaptic ones (particularly from the dorsal hypothalamus). RF stimulation *facilitated* conduction between the hypothalamus and the HC. So Feldman drew up this scheme:

(1) The RF depresses the afferent inflow to the thalamus and to hypothalamus.

(2) The RF potentiates the afferent inflow from thalamus to isocortex and from hypothalamus to archicortex (HC).

(3) The HC depresses the afferent RF–hypothalamic inflow and the neocortex depresses the afferent RF–thalamic inflow.

This suggests that the function that the thalamic specific nuclei subserve with respect to the neocortex (and RF) are subserved by the hypothalamus with respect to the archicortex (HC) and to the RF. One main difference may be that the RF–HC relationship seems to be mainly one of mutual inhibition. Cowan et al (1965) point out that each area of the forebrain is related to a subcortical integrating centre which could be a site for interaction for impulses from the cortex and diencephalic centres:

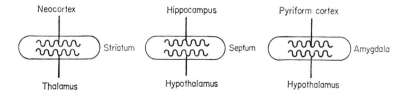

4.4 Seizure activity

The mode of propagation of electrical seizure activity offers important clues for possible functional connections in the brain. This evidence has been taken into account in chapter 2 where these connections were discussed. In general such activity propagates readily from HC and amygdala. Little functional disability seems to result so long as the activity is confined to one HC or amygdala. As soon as it spreads to involve other subcortical structures or temporal lobe cortex, the clinical symptoms of a temporal lobe seizure develop. These HC and amygdala seizures propagate widely to basal forebrain, brainstem, temporal lobe cortex and to the opposite HC or amygdala and to each other.

Cortical epileptic lesions disrupt CRs but only to the stimulus modality concerned and only in the case of new learning—well-established CRs are not affected. Some electrophysiological suggestions as to how this is effected will be discussed in the next section. Patients with centrecephalic lesions do badly on tests requiring sustained vigilance (as might be expected on account of the relationship of these regions to attention) and patients with temporal lobe lesions do badly in tests for memory (as again might be expected).

Chapter 5

THE LIMBIC SYSTEM, CONDITIONED REFLEXES AND LEARNING

5.1 The various stages of conditioned reflex formation

It has become increasingly evident that the limbic system is concerned not only with emotion and the higher control of the internal environment, but also with learning, conditioned reflexes and the higher control of behaviour with respect to the external environment and with matching the 'needs' of the internal environment with the complex details of the actualities and potentialities of the external environment. The interconnected problems of memory, learning and conditioned reflexes may best be approached perhaps by considering what happens when an animal attends to a stimulus and then learns an appropriate reaction towards it (a CR). Seven stages in this reaction have been recognized, each with particular behavioural and/or electrical features: the response configuration:

(1) to a wholly novel stimulus (S);

(2) to the repeated presentation of S without reinforcement:

(3) to the initial reinforcement;

(4) with the first appearance of the CR;

(5) with the optimum level of performance of the CR;

(6) with the development of differentiation between reinforced Ss and non-reinforced Ss and finally;

(7) with the extinction of the CR.

5.1 AROUSAL

Taking these stages in turn the first is concerned with arousal. This is associated in electrical terms with widespread cortical and HC EEG desynchronization. During this phase the potentials evoked by sensory stimulation are large and spread widely all over the cortex. The arousal value of a stimulus is not necessarily related to its intensity but rather to its significance to the individual in that particular context. Thus even before this first behavioural reaction of the organism the sensory inflow from the stimulus must be received, coded, classified, compared and interpreted by the brain (e.g. 'quite novel stimulus' ∴ *alert*: 'bark of dog far off' ∴ *alert*: 'bark of dog very near' ∴ *panic stations*: 'cry of baby' ∴ *alert*: 'only a car passing' ∴ no alert). This activity must involve the entire cortex and the controlling structure would appear to be the mesencephalic RF. The large and widespread evoked potentials in the cortex presumably express this process of classifying and interpreting, etc. proceeding as widely and efficiently as possible. Key (1965) presents evidence to suggest that the amplitude of the secondary surface positive waves, rather than the primary waves, is more clearly related to the level of significance of the stimulus.

John and Killam (1959) using a flickering light as the CS for a CAR response observed high-voltage frequency specific responses to the first presentation of the CS in visual cortex, lateral geniculate body and superior colliculus, and hippocampus. Some following also occurred in amygdala, septum and RF. These quickly habituated without reinforcement in the order: amygdala; RF and superior colliculus; visual cortex; thalamic relay nuclei.

5.1.2 THE ORIENTING RESPONSE

The next development is a complex of motor behaviour known as the 'orienting response'. The animal turns its head and eyes towards the source of the stimulus, pricks up its ears and there are some autonomic changes. The whole response is clearly designed to gather the maximum possible information about S and to set the autonomic scene for any possible flight, fright, or other reaction that may be required. The response is made to an S which is familiar to some, even if only to a very slight degree, but whose meaning is undetermined. A wholly novel stimulus tends to give a 'startle response' where the emphasis is on immediate self-preservation rather than on gathering more information. This is clearly of survival benefit to the organism.

The orienting response can be induced by stimulation of the mesencephalic RF or hypothalamus and can be abolished by lesions of the RF or its pathway to the HC via septum and fornix. During this phase the non-specific thalamic nuclei (code ILTN) with their more localized cortical connections come progressively into action. They serve to localize attention to the cortical areas that turn out to be specifically concerned with the S and to 'switch off' those cortical areas not specifically concerned. This is accompanied by a diminution and change of form of the cortical evoked potentials outside the primary projection area concerned— a reduction taking place particularly in the long-latency polyphasic secondary potentials. The prominent HC rhythm at this stage probably indicates HC inactivity since HC stimulation at this stage abolishes the orientation response.

If the stimuli are repeated and are not reinforced the evoked responses gradually die out,* last of all from layer 4 of the specific sensory cortex involved. The orienting response and the HC theta rhythm (except from the dendritic zones of the central part of the pyramidal cell layer) also disappear. S, not conveying anything of interest or importance to the organism, ceases to attract attention or have 'meaning' (or potential meaning) and ceases to have much effect on the brain.

Thus the initial stage of response to a stimulus is general *arousal* associated with a cortically mediated evaluation of the significance of S to the organism. This function is largely under the control of the mesencephalic RF with its widespread sensing in flow and cortical connections. If the S is (probably/possibly) significant, but its precise meaning is undetermined, the orienting response develops marked by inhibition of HC activity (by the mesen-

---

* 'We have *never* seen any sign of habituation in human *primary* sensory cortex, even after thousands of monotonous stimuli. (This is with intracortical electrodes—again the scalp EEG is contaminated by non-specific components which of course do habituate.)' (Grey Walter, 1965).

cephalic RF) and the activation of the mechanisms of selective attention in the thalamic RF (ILTN).

5.1.3 EARLY SIGNS OF CONDITIONING AND INHIBITION

If a stimulus to which habituation had been developed is now reinforced by associating it in time with either reward (e.g. food) or punishment (e.g. an electric shock) it evokes anew behavioural arousal, cortical desynchronization and HC slow waves. The widespread cortical evoked potentials return and get progressively localized, as conditioning proceeds to the cortical region of the *unconditioned* stimulus. However, it must be noted that these particular electrical signs are not necessary for conditioned reflexes to develop, as this can occur in their absence as under atropine.

As we have seen Adey is of the opinion that the HC theta rhythm has a more interesting function than merely indicating that the HC is out of action. He feels that it is associated with the execution of a planned sequence of behaviour, in this case with approach behaviour towards a food reward. In his experiments the pre-approach record showed a wide spectrum of activity around 3–4 c/s; but when the animal actually approached the food tray the characteristic HC theta rhythm of around 6 c/s became apparent. By computer analysis techniques he has shown that the phase relationships of the theta waves show highly consistent patterns in varying circumstances. For example, when the animal made the appropriate response to the task set the waves from the dorsal HC led those from the entorhinal area by a constant factor of as much as 30 m.sec. This phase relationship was reversed if an incorrect response was made. As training proceeded a 6 c/s rhythm developed in primary sensory and sensorimotor cortex and in the RF and these became progressively more locked in frequency with the HC rhythm. Then again, in *early* training, the main afferent inflow to the HC followed the path septum–fornix–dentate gyrus–HC. In the fully trained animal this flow seemed to be reversed and this pathway became efferent from the HC rather than afferent to it.

Grastyán (1960) supports the contention that the HC theta rhythm indicates 'inhibition'. He supposes that the function of the HC in this context is to inhibit the orienting reflex mediated by the RF—that is to prevent its manifestation. Therefore if approach activity is to follow in the orienting response the HC must come back into action. As conditioning proceeds the CS leads directly to the CR without any intervening orienting reflex. The animal goes directly to the food box on hearing the buzzer. It 'knows the meaning' of S. In this case the CS gives immediate HC desynchronization without any theta rhythm appearing. Grastyán claims that, as the HC theta rhythm occurs during approach behaviour, the HC is not inhibiting this particular aspect of the 'orienting' function of the RF. This seems perhaps a fine point as to when one type of behaviour gives over to another during a continuous sequence of actions. Adey's results suggest, however, that the role of the HC is more complex; that it plays a part in evaluating the correctness of the response and that its mode of response is affected by the degree of training reached.

The relationship of the HC theta rhythm to meaning is illustrated by the following experiment. An alimentary CR to an S was built up to the degree that no orienting response and no HC theta rhythm was any longer obtainable. If the same S was now presented in a novel situation (e.g. not in the familiar feed box but in another one), the HC theta rhythm and the alerting response returned (i.e. 'familiar S but what does it mean in here?'). Clearly the mechanisms computing the significance of S do so with respect to the total environmental situation.

Conditioning is accompanied by other changes in the cortex. A CR may be set up by using an electrical stimulus (e.g. to the motor cortex producing limb movement) as the UCS and an auditory or visual S as the CS. After sufficient presentations the sound alone will elicit the movement. During this procedure there is a widespread fall in thresholds in the motor cortex for eliciting movements by local electrical stimulation. As the CR becomes established these thresholds rise except at the locus of reinforcement (corresponding to Pavlov's 'consolidation' and 'inhibition'). At the sites of Pavlovian inhibition slow waves are alleged to appear in the

EEG. A stimulus undergoing conditioning acts less and less on the general arousal mechanism of the midbrain RF and more and more on very localized areas of the thalamic RF. The actual 'closure' or completion of the CR does not go from the CS cortical centre directly to the UCS cortical centre because it is not abolished by cutting these direct paths. It goes via the RF mainly in the thalamus; hypothalamic mechanisms may also be involved (figs. 20, 21).

Morrell (1961) also suggests that slow waves may not merely indicate 'inhibition' but that they may subserve a 'regenerating mechanism' that imprints a record of the experience. But he goes on to point out that in all learning there is a logical need for the transient obliteration of homeostatic regulation mechanisms that would themselves tend to counteract any change.

External inhibition (i.e. the inhibition of a CR by a competing external stimulus) is associated with cortical synchronization, and internal inhibition (due to extinction or differentiation of a CR) is associated with hypersynchronous slow waves in the EEG. These slow waves are seen during the extinction of a CR (when the S is no longer reinforced and thus loses meaning), and during a forced delay between a CS and its correlated CR and in response to the non-reinforced member of a pair of differentiated stimuli. However, the form of the response depends much on the meaning of S. In a situation where S means 'no shock' slow waves appear in the EEG (i.e. relax: see also 5.16). In a situation where the same S signifies 'food', an alert EEG pattern results.

5.1.4 THE ROLE OF STEADY POTENTIALS

Another electrical technique that has been used in this field has been the study of steady potentials. The ordinary nerve impulse is a dynamic affair but much of the brain's work seems to be carried out by the maintenance of steady potential differences between different loci. If a direct current is applied to the motor cortex (anodal polarization) this gives rise to a motor response in the appropriate part of the body whenever any sensory stimulus (above a certain threshold) is applied. The motor cortex has become as it were sensitized. If now the current is switched off the motor cortex will still react in this way but only to those sensory stimuli that had been given during the period of current flow. A learned response has been set up in this way and the part of the cortex wherein this altered behaviour 'resides' is called a 'dominant locus'.

These dominant loci can also reroute signals in the CNS. The development of a conditioned reflex clearly demands some re-routing of signals and the problem arises of how this is done. These steady potentials and dominant loci may supply some of the answer. If, for example, (i) a familiar auditory or visual S is given, no change of heart rate or respiration results. If, however, they are given while anodal polarization is applied to the hypo-thalamus, cardiac and respiratory changes ensue. Then again (ii) one can establish a CR with some motor response such as lifting a paw. If the CS is now given during anodal polarization of the hypothalamus, the somatic motor response is abolished and autonomic responses appear instead.

There is further evidence that these dominant loci do play some part in normal physiology and are not mere artifacts. If one stimulates the centromedian nucleus of the thalamus a $\frac{1}{2}$–1 mV DC shift appears in the central ipsilateral cortex. These DC shifts can be conditioned and, as mentioned above, stimulation of this nucleus can evoke a pre-established CR. Stimulation here can also interfere with learning a CAR (presumably by 'jamming') but has no effect on the retention of a pre-established CAR. These short-term circuits can maintain temporary connections and re-routing of signals. The length of time that anodally polarized cells can store information is similar to the time course of memory that is sensitive to ECT or concussion in rat and man. Furthermore all physical agents that induce amnesia (concussion, ECT, etc.) also induce significant steady potential shifts. Epileptic foci are also marked by standing potentials in the absence of seizures and these foci disrupt the formation of CRs in the surrounding cortex. These potentials may contribute to the symptomatology of epilepsy.

An interrelationship between the HC theta rhythm and DC potentials is reported by Parmeggiani and Rabini (1964). The

DC shifts produced in the cortex by stimulation of the sciatic are greatly reduced by coagulation of the septum, which abolishes theta.

The role that such DC changes may play in human voluntary action has been suggested by Grey Walter et al (1964). His subjects were subjected to the following experiment. A flash (conditional stimulus) was followed at a constant interval by a series of clicks. A flash alone, or a series of clicks alone, causes an evoked potential in the frontal lobe. If, however, the subject is told to press a button whenever he hears the clicks (imperative stimulus), then the evoked potential of the 'warning' flash is followed by a large negative DC potential that Grey Walter has called the 'contingent negative variation' (CNV). The amplitude of this potential is directly proportional to the contingency of the association between the two stimuli. That is to say, if only some of the flashes are followed by clicks the amplitude of the CNV falls. The CNV responds to verbal instruction as it does not appear if the subject is told in advance there would be no flashes.

This phenomenon is similar in some respect to the effects of anodol (positive) polarization of the motor cortex (already described). In that case, it will be recalled, the organism responds to any sensory stimulus presented during the period of polarization by movement of the part related to the area of the motor cortex stimulated. For the 15 minutes or so it responds only to those stimuli that were presented during the period of polarization. In the present case the polarization is *negative* and this 'primes' the cortex to respond to a particular stimulus to produce movement. The respective roles of negative and positive polarization during single S–R reactions as well as more complex conditioning reactions would seem to offer an interesting field of study.

Lippold and Redfearn (1964) have reported interesting changes in mood produced by polarizing the frontal cortex in conscious human subjects by using small direct currents. Positive polarization induces 'an elevation of mood and an increased involvement in the environment; scalp-negative current flow produces withdrawal and quietness'.

Kawamura et al (1967) have reported that the DC potential

across a rabbit's skull shifts during eating and drinking (in opposite senses). The changes were thought to be due to changes in the potential of the blood–brain barrier following changes in the osmotic pressure of the plasma. DC potential changes accompany arousal from sleep (Wurtz, 1965). In self-stimulation and avoidance experiments in rats (Wurtz, 1966) arousal produced a surface negative DC shift. A second smaller shift was seen that appeared to be related to the reinforcing effect of the S. There was a tendency for negative shifts to be associated with Ss and positive ones with escape. The mechanism of production of these DC shifts in the cortex have been ascribed to polarized gradients between the ends of highly laminated cortical neurones. But stimulation of the RF produces DC shifts in the posterior hypothalamus (as well as the sensorimotor cortex) and the neurones in the former region lack any such laminated structure. The cells are embedded in a random fashion in a dense neuropil that runs in all directions. Hence the DC shifts are more probably due to local synaptic change such as IPSPs (Hayward et al, 1966).

5.1.5 CHANGES IN IMPEDANCE

Another parameter of neuronal function that has been measured is the impedance (electrical resistance) of parts of the brain. Falls in impedance have been noted in cortical areas during learning in a T-maze. At early stages of learning a transient fall took place. At high performance levels a deeper fall occurred that began immediately following the presentation of the test and persisted until the completion of the task. This was followed by a slow rise and a return to normality in 6–8 seconds. Adey supposes that these impedance shifts may arise from movements of ionic material between various tissue compartments of the CNS—intraneural, intraglial and extracellular. These impedance shifts may arise particularly from glial cells which may act not merely as purveyors of nutriment to neurones but may possibly have functions in information storage and as modulators of electronic processes in dendrites, determining aspects of both their rate and rhythmicity. Grey Walter (1965) comments, however:

'We here are very sceptical about the interpretation of *impedance measurements* in the brain. There are so many sources of variation that one must really prove in each case what a change is due to. Local oxygen tension controls the impedance of noble metal electrodes (and stainless steel). The pH is also important. The proportion of CSF, blood, gray matter, white matter in any region determines the basic impedance (in resistive units the R of CSF < blood < gray matter < white matter). The impedance of an oxygen electrode falls with activity since this produces more CO_2 which dilates the blood vessels etc. Flicker increases O_2a (lowers impedance of gold electrode) and increases blood flow in area 17 but not 18 or 19. Reading or looking at pictures increases O_2a in 18 and 19 as well, provided the pictures are 'interesting'.

We have made a survey of impedance at 1 kc/s of 68 electrodes in a patient's brain. Both R and C vary by factors of 2–8 and without relation to position or other features.'

5.1.6 THE DIFFERENTIATION OF CONDITIONED REFLEXES

The differentiation of a CR follows a definite pattern as well. For example, a CR can be established using a flickering light as the CS. If then a light flickering at another frequency is presented the evoked response recurs in regions of the cortex where it had lapsed in response to the first frequency. As these evoked potentials 'follow' the rate of flicker of the light (by having the same frequency), this gives us a useful 'tracer' for the origin and propagation of various electrical patterns of the brain. In the particular experiment described the evoked response occurs at the new frequency at the primary sensory cortex but at the old frequency at the motor cortex.

An animal can be trained to avoid a light flickering at one frequency (if this is associated with shock) and to approach a light flickering at another frequency (if this signifies 'food'). In each case the frequency of the responses evoked in the primary sensory cortex, in the non-specific relay system and the various limbic areas agrees with the stimulus frequency if the animal makes the correct response. But if it makes the wrong response (i.e. approaches an 'avoid' S) the frequency of the responses in the primary sensory cortex will be that of the actual S whereas the frequency in the other areas (including the limbic system) will be that appropriate to the response actually performed (i.e. the frequency of the other S). This suggests that the electrical pattern in these areas is associated in some way with the programme of instruction for the motor performance. This will be discussed further below.

5.1.7 THE EXTINCTION OF A CONDITIONED RESPONSE

Lissák and Grastyán (1957) postulate that there are two different types of mechanism effecting inhibition: (a) in the case of differential inhibition (where one stimulus selectively gains meaning at the expense of another) he supposes that reciprocal inhibitory mechanisms of the brainstem and hypothalamus predominate and (b) in the case of extinction (where an S ceases to have meaning because it is no longer reinforced) he supposes that the HC may be involved. The reciprocal nature of these brainstem mechanisms is evidenced by the fact that stimulation of loci in the RF or hypothalamus which facilitate one CR, invariably inhibit other(s). Behavioural differential inhibition is accompanied, as we saw, by cortical desynchronization and no slow waves are to be observed. Extinction, on the other hand, is associated with cortical slow waves: stimulation of the HC depresses CRs and this is accompanied by cortical slow waves.

5.2 The role of different brain mechanisms in learning

5.2.1 THE ROLE OF THE NEOCORTEX

The discussion so far gives us an indication of how certain aspects of learning and CR formation may be associated with specific brain structures, in particular with the RF, the hypothalamus and the HC. Very crude CRs can be established in a decerebrate animal so the basic mechanism must be present in the diencephalon. Removal of the auditory cortex in animals does not prevent

I

discrimination between simple tones but only between more complex signals. In a case where a tone is the CS bilateral resection of the auditory cortex does not usually abolish the CR nor prevent simple new ones from being formed. Removal of other parts of the cortex outside the areas for the CS and UCS only affects the most complex and delicate discriminations. Removal of the cortex related to the UCS, however, usually markedly impairs the CR. If the entire cortex is removed the animal no longer shows a classical CR to pain (e.g. withdrawal of paw) but it still shows affective and autonomic reactions. These are, however, easily extinguished by failing to reinforce the CS even only on one or two occasions. Thus the major role of neocortex in conditioned reflexes seems to be concerned mainly with the parameter of *complexity*. The dependence of CRs on the cortex related to the UCS may reflect the fact that this cortex is necessary for the motor or autonomic consequences of the CR to appear.

5.2.2 THE ROLE OF SUBCORTICAL STRUCTURES

We have already reviewed much evidence that indicates the involvement of limbic structures in CR formation. Stimulation of points in the RF (midbrain or thalamic) and the hypothalamus may facilitate or inhibit CRs, or may facilitate one and inhibit another CR, or may induce one or another response according to the circumstances. Stimulation of these structures may also interfere with learning (by 'jamming', or by inducing competing emotions, sensations and reactions as well as, possibly, by some direct effect on the learning process *per se*). Partial lesions of the hypothalamus or RF can abolish an alimentary CR (e.g. salivation to sound) while leaving the UCR (in this case salivation when food is placed in the mouth) intact.

Further evidence of the role of subcortical structure comes from experiments, already described, carried out by John and Killam (1959). The CS was a flickering light that gave a 'tracer' stimulus to the brain. They then took recordings from different parts of the brain at different stages of the learning process. During the early stages the still neutral S gave a response mainly in specific sensory structures and HC: some in RF, septum and amygdala. When the conditional emotional response is developing (S indicates 'shock coming') but no CAR learned yet, these signals are rerouted—presumably by the mechanism that computes the S–shock association probability. This causes the specific waves to diminish in the lateral geniculate body and the rhythm now appears in the RF–septal–HC complex, but not in the amygdala. As soon as the animal has developed an effective motor procedure to avoid the shock the response again returns to the specific sensory system and the responses in the other two loci die away, except for a new rhythm in the amygdala—the 40 c/s rhythm.

Another experiment gave a further indication of the possible role of subcortical mechanisms. A differential response was conditioned to 10 c/s flash ('food') and a 6 c/s flash ('no food'). The animal then received a long series of 6 c/s stimuli, and then was switched suddenly to 10 c/s. At the moment of change the new 'environmental' rhythm appeared in the midbrain RF and the visual isocortex whereas the 6 c/s rhythm still appeared in the records from the HC and the thalamic RF. As soon as the animal 'woke up' to the new situation and responded correctly to the new S (by going to the food box) the HC wave went and the thalamic RF rhythm switched to 10 c/s. This suggests that the electrical activity of the HC and the thalamic RF (modulated in this fashion by the 'old' 6 c/s S) is concerned with the immediate memory to which the animal is responding, or even that it may carry an executive programme associated with matching behaviour with the state of the environment. Thus, during certain stages of learning, the CNS can produce an internal rhythm similar to that which it is 'expecting'. In a later tracer experiment (Lindsley et al, 1968) the Ss were two different shapes, both illuminated by light flickering at 10 c/s, one signifying 'food', the other 'no food'. During learning the 10 c/s rhythm appeared in the visual pathways, RF and various thalamic areas with less striking labelling seen in the ventromedial nucleus of the thalamus and the MFB. It was *not* seen in the HC or the amygdala. The latter showed bursts of 40 c/s rhythm when the task became difficult. During incorrect responses the 10 c/s rhythm was much less well marked and could be absent. Atropine led to a 'fragmentation of the appropriate sequences of behavior; this fragmenting led to long latence responses and finally failure to respond'. The exact role of these HC and thalamic RF rhythms has been subject to some dispute. Some people have suggested that the information that 'S is a 10 c/s rhythm' is carried by the fact that the nucleus concerned is producing a 10 c/s rhythm itself. However, Deutsch (1962) has criticized this idea on the basis (i) that frequencies of S can be discriminated well outside the range that the EEG can follow and (ii) that frequency discrimination can be effected by means of tuned nerve nets, according to elementary electronic principles, without the necessity of having the nervous system play over a copy of it. The problem of what sort of information cerebral rhythms can carry seems to be a very complex one (see e.g. Adey, 1967; Freeman, 1963). The appearance of the rhythm in these brain loci may merely indicate the activation of these loci and the rhythm is a functionally unimportant byproduct of this activity that carries no code function but results merely from the impress of (modulation by) the form of the original stimulus pattern. Morrell (1961) suggests that the appearance of a specific rhythm in a nucleus may mean (i) that the nucleus is now more 'excitable' or in a phase of liability to synchronous activity and therefore more likely to be driven by an externally applied rhythm; (ii) the information may not be carried by a crude comparison of frequency but by subtle patterns of phase relationship. 'Attention has been drawn to the dubious role of "tracer signals" in analysis of ongoing activity in the central nervous system. In most instances they are within the frequency bands that characterize spontaneous activity in the area. Moreover, there is very great difficulty in deciding whether a sequence of polyphasic potentials, constituting an evoked potential, are a measure of a local process triggered by a single afferent volley, or whether they represent a continued synaptic input which in turn is inducing recurrent postsynaptic events. The distinction is critical to any argument about the role of the evoked potential. In the informational sense, we are dealing with a multidimensional signal space, partly occupied by internal "housekeeping" events, and also concerned with afferent information in modalities that may relate strictly to the conditioning process. Some at least of the evoked potential studies have introduced irrelevant transients into such a complexly operating system, so that changes in their configuration can have little merit in measuring the status of the tissue as it relates to the conditioning process. This would appear to relate particularly to the size of an evoked auditory potential in a cat that is orienting to a visual stimulus such as a mouse' (Adey, 1965). Adey has shown that a frequency modulation is present in the 6 c/s HC rhythm at moments of maximum attention. Such modulation would serve to increase the information carrying capacity of the rhythm; (iii) the information may be carried by discrete action potentials carried over axons rather than the largely dendritic EEG rhythms which serve some ancillary function in this case. As Jasper et al (1958) say '... the waves themselves ... are not caused by the grouped firing of individual neurones since they continue after cell discharge has been arrested by anaesthesia. They seem to be of the nature of dendritic potentials which modulate, facilitate or inhibit the discharge of cortical cells. Inferences regarding excitatory or inhibitory states in relation to behaviour or to mechanisms of conditioning based on changes in surface electrical activity must be tentative until confirmed by records of the firing of cortical cells detected only with microelectrodes'. The independence between CR behaviour and its electrical concomitants (as under the effect of atropine) has already been mentioned. Adey (1965) suggests that computer techniques might reveal relationships between EEG phenomena and behaviour under atropine. Features of the electrical rhythms induced by the stimuli may also play a part in this sort of experiment. For example, some cats were trained to avoid a 4 c/s stimulus and others to approach a 10 c/s stimulus. Then electrical stimuli at these two frequencies were applied direct to the brain in both series of cats. In both the 4 c/s rhythm S was much more effective in suppressing the CR, although the 'meaning' of this rhythm was different in the two groups. It is also apparent that the precise physical properties of the electrical stimulus are very important in determining its effects.

There is some evidence that food reflexes and avoidance

reactions are mediated in part by different mechanisms. For example, a frequency specific response induced in the RF and HC is depressed by the establishment of a CAR but not by an alimentary CR. Again, if animals are trained to associate shock with one stimulus and food reward with another, and then are placed in the environment where shock is expected, they show sustained cortical desynchronization and no response to the alimentary CS. Indeed they often give an erroneous avoidance reaction to it. If they are now given chlorpromazine the previously dominant CAR is abolished. The defensive CS now gives cortical desynchronization and the alimentary CR. Thus the chlorpromazine has knocked out the defensive reaction without affecting the alimentary one.

Chapter 6

MECHANISMS OF MEMORY

One of the major problems outstanding in neurobiology is the mechanism of storage of memory in the brain. It has generally been agreed for many years that our memories and skills are stored in some physical form in the brain and the term 'engram' was coined to describe this.

A host of clinical and experimental facts have suggested that there are basically two types of memory in the brain—a *labile recent memory*, and a *constant permanent memory*. The classical mechanism proposed runs something like this: The incoming sensory stimuli set up patterns of activity in the brain based on feed-back loops and closed circuits. These can maintain the memory for a few minutes after which the reverberating activity gradually dies away. Permanent memory formation depends somehow on the change in the property of individual synapses, so that a synapse frequently used tends to develop some change in its properties, which entail that the next time the stimulus is presented, the cells that fired previously will tend to fire again. Thus, in summary, the classical theory supposes that short-term memory depends on activity in nerve nets and long-term memory depends on some alteration in synaptic knobs caused thereby.

The effect of ECT upon memory was advanced as evidence in support of this hypothesis. If a rat is given something simple to learn, and immediately afterwards is given ECT, it fails to learn. The usual experiment is to set up a passive conditioned avoidance response by electrifying its food box and giving it a shock when it goes to eat. Normally this leads to a prolonged avoidance of the food box—but if this experience is followed in a few seconds by an ECT the rat will approach the food box, when it recovers, in obvious forgetfulness of the painful shock it received the last time.

This explanation fitted in nicely with the concept of the massive flow of electricity through the brain wiping out all activity in the postulated nerve nets.

However, some recent experiments have thrown doubt on this account. One experiment (Misanin et al, 1968) was conducted as follows: The shock from the electrified food box, followed by ECT, led to amnesia for the shock the next day. The memory could be recalled, however, merely by giving the rat on the second day an electric shock to its paw as a 'reminder'. In another experiment (Misanin et al, 1968) a conditioned avoidance response to a specific sensory stimulus was set up in a group of rats. Immediate ECT in twenty rats produced the usual amnesia. Then the next day forty rats were presented briefly with the CS. Then one-half received ECT within a few seconds and the rest did not. Twenty further rats received only ECT. The rats that received ECT following on reactivation of the memory trace showed subsequent amnesia, whereas neither of the other two groups did so. Thus the authors concluded that ECT does not produce amnesia only for recent events, but it also depends on the state of the memory trace at the time. 'Thus, it appears that a primary determinant of amnesia is that the memory-trace system must be in a state of change at the time of ECT.'

A third important experiment was carried out by Nielson (1968). He detailed three currently held theories why ECT interferes with memory:

 (i) by interference with reverberating circuits
(ii) by inducing fear and
(iii) by conditioned inhibition.

The results of a long series of experiments provided evidence against all three theories and in favour of a fourth. He points out that the 'amnesia' produced by ECT for recent events is temporary anyway and the return of memory is hastened if the increased motor activity produced by ECT is prevented. Secondly ECT produces a charge in the physical property of the brain. Electrical stimulation of the brain can be used as a CS for a conditioned avoidance response. ECT raises the threshold for this stimulus some five-fold, and this takes some 4 days to return to normal.

If this change in brain excitability is controlled for by using previous ECT so that the *learning* of the conditioned response and its *recall* are carried out in similar conditions of brain excitability, then ECT does not lead to any amnesia at all.

In other words Nielson claims that the amnesia following ECT is really an example of state-dependent learning. The classical example of the phenomenon is that a conditioned reflex established under the effect of a particular drug—e.g. strychnine—can only be activated subsequently following the injection of strychnine. ECT appears to be acting in exactly the same way except that the factor that must be kept constant for memory to be recalled properly is a physical property—excitability—rather than purely chemical. Thus these workers claim that ECT interferes with the *recall of memory* as the classical theory claimed.

If we now turn to the mechanism laying down permanent memory, this is certainly more complex than the simple scheme the classical theory suggests. Many people have pointed out that the mere use of a learning system leads not to learning but to habituation. Thus the mechanism of reinforcement and emotional mechanism must play an important role in consolidation of memory.

A great deal of interest has been shown recently in the concept that protein synthesis is involved in engram formation. The experimental basis for this lies in the effect of inhibitors of protein synthesis such as puromycin and acetoxycycloheximide on learning. The former is not a good compound to use as it causes epileptiform disturbances in the hippocampus and these might be the proximate cause of the memory disruption. The latter, however, does not. Barondes and Cohen (1968) report that acetoxycycloheximide will disrupt memory formation but it must be present in the brain at the time of the presentation of the stimulus or given immediately (up to 5 minutes) afterwards. In this case the rats learned as well as saline-injected controls, remembered the conditioned response normally for 3 hours but had almost entirely forgotten it by 6 hours and the amnesia persisted when tested again 7 days later. That is the inhibition of protein synthesis affects permanent memory and not recent memory, but it must be present at the time the S is given or very shortly thereafter.

We will return later to the problem of how protein synthesis could act in the consolidation of memory.

The role of acetyl choline in memory formation

The roles of cholinergic systems in memory formation have been explored by Deutsch and his co-workers. They found that a well-learned task is blocked by the anticholinesterase DFP whereas this drug enhanced poorly learned tasks. Likewise, in a given learning trial, a low dose of DFP enhanced learning and a higher dose inhibited learning (Deutsch and Lutsky, 1967). The time course of the learning situation was also important. DFP produced no, or only weak, amnesia for tasks learned 0–3 days before, but considerable amnesia for habits learned 5–14 days before. They therefore supposed that '... the effective physiological basis of memory is a change in synaptic conductance, mediated by an increase in the concentration of effective transmitter, in this instance probably acetyl choline'. Scopolamine had the reverse effect to DFP (Deutsch and Rocklin, 1967). Thus DFP is supposed to facilitate the poorly learned memory by protecting the acetyl choline from breakdown and to block the overlearned memory by inducing excessive depolarization blockade. The acetyl choline mechanism could well be part of the recall system. However, Richardson and Glow (1967) found that DFP appeared to act in their experiments by reducing the accuracy of the performance rather than the ability to carry out sensory discrimination. For example, increasing the cost of making errors (e.g. by introducing shock) restored normal performance.

They noted that the animals were half paralysed by DFP and attribute some of the apparent diminution of learning to the gross motor disability.

Excess water and salt in the body, produced by manipulating antidiuretic hormone, can function as a drive and return to normal levels produced by any external consummatory act can function as a reward (Miller et al, 1968). Removal of the posterior and intermediate lobe of the pituitary facilitates the rate of extinction of a conditioned response. This was shown not to be due to any disturbance of water metabolism nor depression of ACTH release. The depression of conditioned behaviour could be prevented by the peptides ACTH, pitressin and vasopressin. De Weld (1965) concludes: 'The marked behavioural effects of the pituitary peptides, as shown by the present experiments, focus a possible physiological function on these and other peptides in the central nervous system.'

An assumption that we have held for years is that no new neurones are developed in the brain after birth and that a newborn child has its full complement of neurones The subsequent growth of the brain has been ascribed to myelination, growth of glia, etc. However, Altman (1967) has shown recently that this is not so at all. Neurones certainly do not divide, but new neurones are formed after birth from the ependyma. In fact the neurones of the newborn are remarkably different from those of the adult.

The newborn human has its full complement of large pyramidal cells but their dendrites and spine systems are not fully developed. The thalamocortical endings are also rather simple, there is little myelination, and only a few small interneurones.

During the first 2 years of life the dendrites sprout many branches and these develop a fully fledged spine apparatus. The ependymal cells continue to divide and give rise to neuroblasts which migrate through the cortex to become the granule cells and other small cells. As these small cells migrate they pass through the dentritic fields of macroneurons to which they attach their axons as they pass. This cell and dendrite proliferation is under environmental control.

These findings emphasize the importance of the early environment on later psychological development. For certain noxious early environmental situations could well result in the establishment of certain patterns of neural growth and connections that will tend to lead to malfunction later on. Thus the wiring pattern in the brain may be quite different in different people and the causes for the differences may be traced to the environment. Rats raised in an enriched environment, as compared with rats raised in an impoverished one, have heavier brains, which is due entirely to growth of the cerebral cortex and the hippocampus

(Diamond et al, 1964; Rosenzweig, 1966). Different cortical areas can be selectively developed by manipulating different aspects of the environment. AChE increases particularly in the cortex, but number of cells per unit field falls—so the growth may be mainly dendrites glia. Even so simple a procedure as rearing rats in cages with black-striped rats versus plain white rats induces significant changes (Singh et al, 1967). There were no changes in total protein or RNA.

An important study has recently been carried out by Meissner (1968) on the Korsakoff psychosis. The usual picture one has of the nature of Korsakoff's psychosis is that it involves somehow a defect in laying down permanent memories, although Korsakoff himself thought the defect was one of recall. One also tends to think of the permanent memory store as some kind of simple container in which memories are put, rather like the memory tape of a computer. But as we suggested above memory may be much more complex than this.

Meissner made an extensive study of the condition using many tests and has claimed there are two basic disabilities: (i) A tendency to limited or fragmentary impressions isolated from the flow of experience. (ii) A rigidity and inflexibility of originally adopted sets.

All tests for memory are affected. (i) Patients acquire less information and forget it faster. (ii) New associations form but dissolve rapidly. (iii) There is no relearning.

Their learning is based on immediate cues and they can handle tasks involving only one or two items quite well.

As soon as the number of items goes beyond three they are lost. Particular difficulties are experienced in tasks when sequential activities are required. They cannot do tasks involving the retention of information for later application in planned action.

He classified memories as follows:

Primary memory. Simple with not more than two items to be related: the elements are either transferred to secondary memory or are displaced by new inputs. It depends on septal–HC circuits.

Secondary memory. The new input from the primary memory is consolidated by rehearsal. New input is stored by a complex coding and integrating mechanism which requires the function of sequential organization in the efficient storage and recall of memory. Active retrieval requires the effective operation of sequencing mechanisms. 'Recall of complex events requires a constructive sequential reorganization of stored elements which enables the mind to reconstruct impressions in a contextually organized fashion.' This function is disrupted in Korsakoff's psychosis. It depends on temporo-ammonic circuits.

Tertiary memory. (Overlearned.) Elements in tertiary memory have achieved a level of sequential integration and consolidation such that active recall does not require any sequential reconstruction. Material already in the tertiary memory is not affected by Korsakoff's psychosis, but no new material can be added—because any new material must come from the secondary memory. Thus the HC and its circuits could function in the manner of the register of a computor.

Chapter 7

SOME NEUROCHEMICAL
ASPECTS OF BRAIN FUNCTION

The discovery of the specific neurones in the brain that contain biogenic amines (NE, 5HT) by the Swedish workers using fluorescent histochemical methods has resulted in widespread interest in the chemical factors in brain organization, as opposed to the purely morphological and electrical factors that we have been considering in the main until now. The NE neurones have their cell bodies mainly in the locus coerulus in the pons and medulla, with a few scattered in the hypothalamus and midbrain central grey. The 5HT neurones are located almost entirely in the raphe nuclei, also placed in the pons and medulla. The axons of both traverse the MFB and are distributed very widely throughout the brain, including the neocortex. Here very fine axons containing catecholamines may be observed to run through all layers mainly in a vertical direction making long synaptic courses along the apical dendrites of the pyramidal cells with many varicosities en route. The NE content of the cortex is 0·35 μg/g, which is quite high, whereas the dopamine content is very low (Fuxe et al, 1968). It is found in practically all areas and is concentrated in layers 1, 3 and 4. Layers 5 and 6 contain little. The cingulate, insular and frontal regions contain the most. Thus the power to control the widespread release of these two amines is concentrated into two small areas of the brainstem. Lesions of the MFB lower the levels of brain amines rostral to the lesion and have no effect caudal to that level, indicating the upward direction of the traffic. The activity of 5HTP decarboxylase is also reduced. If we enquire into the possible function of these systems, we can note the following.

(1) *Noradrenalin*

Noradrenaline (NE) is widely released in the brain during the sham rage reaction. Eleftheriou and Boehlke (1967) showed that the activity of monoamine oxidase increases for 1–2 days in the hypothalamus in mice following defeat in fight with trained fighter mice. This suggests that the enzyme has been induced to cope with excess amine(s) release. Severe stress (conditioned anxiety, overcrowding, injections of adrenaline) applied to pregnant rats led to permanent changes in the behaviour of their offspring, in this case they became less emotional and fearful; whereas injections of hydrocortisone or NE made the young rats more fearful and emotional. These results were felt to be due to the direct effect of the hormone on the embryo.

Claims have been made that the reward system, closely linked to the MFB, is adrenergic. Poschel and Ninteman (1963) showed that all drugs that raise SS rates modify, either directly or indirectly, the action of NE. Amphetamine potentiates SS rates; imipramine has no effect by itself but potentiates the effect of amphetamine. Pretreatment with drugs like chlorpromazine or α MMT inhibit SS, presumably by their central antiadrenergic effect. It has been reported that rats will also work for cerebral injections of cholinergic agents as well as chelating agents (Olds et al, 1964). However, later results (Domino and Olds, 1968) indicate that SS is inhibited by physostigmine but not by neostigmine. The former raises brain ACh but the latter, not being able to cross the blood–brain barrier, does not. The authors suggest that these results are due to the activation of a cholinergic 'no-go' system complementary to the adrenergic 'go' system. Injections of NE into the dorsal hypothalamus of the rabbit potentiates defensive reflexes and depresses food reflexes for 30 minutes after which these effects reverse. Larger doses induce sleep (Kalynzhugi, 1964).

Stress tends to raise brain amine levels (Nielson and Fleming, 1968). Cold stress raises only the level of DA and foot shock raises both NE and DA. ECT raises amine levels but only in stressed animals. The authors postulate that '. . . changes in brain catecholamine levels may be the mechanisms responsible for the interaction of the stresses produced by the environment with the type of behaviour elicited by the environment'. Thiery et al (1968), however, showed that the significant variable produced by stress is an increase in the *turnover* of NE in the brain. This occurs mainly in the brainstem, mesencephalon and cord but does occur elsewhere as well. There was also an increase in the synthesis of 5HT. Severe stress depresses NE turnover rates. There was no change in DA. Rats with lesions in the amygdala are hypersensitive to amphetamine suggesting a denervation hypersensitivity and so the possibility of an adrenergic efferent pathway from the amygdala concerned in the modulation of emotional responses. NE fibres run in the fornix to synapse on the apical dendrites of the HC pyramids and the basal dendrites of the dentate cells.

A most interesting observation in man was made by Schachter and Singer (1962), who showed the infusions of catecholamines accentuate the particular effect produced by the environment. That is anxiety increased in an anxiety-provoking situation and relaxation was potentiated in a relaxing environment. NE is also closely concerned with sleep, particularly with the REM phase.

(2) *Acetylcholine*

Acetylcholine may be an important central transmitter in the cortex, particularly in layers 2, 3 and 4 (Phillis and York, 1967). There is also a deal of evidence to link ACh with cortical activation (Domino, 1968). There is both biological and chemical evidence of its presence and its levels alter appropriately with changes in function. Likewise its agonists, antagonists and drugs that affect its metabolism, all affect arousal. The septal–HC pathway is cholinergic (Lewis and Shute, 1967) but the main inputs into the HC (the temporo-ammonic, mossy and commissural fibres) are not. The dentate gyrus is particularly rich in AChE. Conduction in the granule cell layer is blocked by 10^{-7} M ACh (possibly due to excessive depolarization) but the synapses on the apical dendrites of these cells in the molecular layer are not affected (Yamamoto and Kawai, 1967). The receptors in the HC seem to be muscarinic in nature (Baker and Benedict, 1968). The HC does not respond to nicotine. In Biscoe and Straughan's experiments (1966) ACh excited some 50 per cent of the cells they tested in the HC, and this effect was blocked by atropine. 5HT mostly depressed cells. Both these effects had a slow time course. Glutamate excited and GABA depressed all cells, both with a rapid time course.

Stumpf (1965) reported that many drugs induce HC theta (e.g. some cholinergic, some adrenergic, nicotine, ether, etc.) but that this is an indirect effect and these drugs act directly on the septum. Nicotine and eserine appear to synchronize septal firing patterns. LSD acts directly on the HC depressing the firing rate of the pyramidal cells.

The main efferent pathway to the mamillary bodies is not cholinergic. But the most important cholinergic pathway is concerned with arousal (RF to cortex). It runs as follows (Shute and Lewis, 1967).

(i) The dorsal tegmental pathway runs from the midbrain tegmentum to the tectum, geniculate bodies and thalamus (particularly the centromedian and intralaminar nuclei, which have a cholinergic neuropil—but the cells are not cholinergic—and the anterior thalamic nucleus).

(ii) The ventral tegmental pathway running to the lateral hypothalamus and to the basal forebrain area where many cells contain ACh.

(iii) Several cholinergic pathways connect between the following—globus pallidus, caudate and all forebrain cortical areas: posterior and lateral hypothalamus and lateral preoptic area with the septum and amygdala. The cholinergic cells in these structures look very like RF cells and Shute and Lewis call the entire system the 'ascending cholinergic reticular system' and feel that it may be equivalent to the physiologically defined ascending reticular activation system responsible for arousal. Phillis (1968) found a widespread release of ACh from the cortex following stimulation of a sensory nerve or of the RF again lending support to the hypothesis that the cortical arousal mechanism is cholinergic. However, Jasper and Koyama (1968) showed that, following RF stimulation, the level of ACh in the prefusate from the cortex went up by some 2–3-fold, but that the level of glutamic acid increased

K

by some 10–20-fold. This suggested that glutamic acid was also a candidate to be the transmitter concerned with cortical arousal.

Injections of carbachol into the caudate nucleus or the ventrolateral nucleus of the thalamus, in low dosage, inhibited bar pressing while the animal remained alert. In higher dosage (with possible diffusion) a rage reaction results with autonomic signs. Dopamine injected into the caudate nucleus produced no behavioural signs (Hall et al, 1968).

THE ROLE OF CHOLINERGIC AND ADRENERGIC MECHANISMS IN THE CONTROL OF EATING AND DRINKING

Much work has been done on the role of NE and ACh in the control of drinking and eating. There is good evidence that the former is controlled by adrenergic and the latter by cholinergic mechanisms. Carbachol injected into the dorsomedial and lateral hypothalamus always induces drinking and injections of NE into the same area always induces eating. However, the situation is not that simple. Carbachol induces, and NE inhibits, drinking when injected into the anterior hypothalamus and preoptic area. But NE will induce drinking if given into the preoptic area during food deprivation, and carbachol inhibits drinking if given into the anterior hypothalamus during water deprivation (Hutchinson and Renfrew, 1967).

Injection of saline into the lateral ventricle of normal rats leads to eating and drinking responses. The former are abolished by lesions of the ventromedial nucleus. Rats with lesions of the lateral hypothalamus are aphagic and adipsic but eventually recover. But they still lack many regulatory functions. They do not respond to hypoglycaemia (induced by insulin) by eating and they do not drink to correct disturbances of body water balance caused by hyperthermia or water deprivation. They cannot compensate for sodium deficiency nor does intracranial carbachol have its usual effect (Baile et al, 1967). Injections into the amygdala of deprived animals were also effective. NE increased food and decreased water intake and ACh had the opposite effect (Singer and Montgomery, 1968).

Contrasting effects of cholinergic and adrenergic stimulation of the hypothalamus are apparent in other areas. Carbachol induces a general fearful reaction from many areas and in larger doses led to attack. Adrenaline led to a drowsy state. Injections of carbachol into the dorsomedial nucleus of the hypothalamus have been reported to give exploratory behaviour, whereas adrenergic stimulation led to playful behaviour (Myers, 1964).

However, species differences may play an important role here. In dog and monkey catecholamines lower and 5HT raises the body temperature, whereas in rabbit and sheep these effects are reversed (Feldberg et al, 1967).

SEROTONIN

An important role of 5HT in the brain is concerned with sleep, particularly slow wave sleep. Another important role is suggested by the fact that the hallucinogenic drugs had been shown to produce their effects by action on the central 5HT mechanisms, mainly of an inhibitory nature. Thus the manifold effect of these drugs may be due in part to the inhibition of the serotonin-based mechanisms in the brain and in part to the unbalanced excessive activity of the adrenergic system. This in turn suggests that mechanisms concerned in the organization of perception, thinking, affect and rational behaviour depend on the proper balance of the NE and 5HT mechanisms, and cholinergic mechanisms, too, since delirium results from blockade of that system by agents such as atropine.

Stimulation of the raphe nuclei leads to a widespread release of serotonin throughout the forebrain (Sheard and Aghajanian, 1968). The behavioural concomitants of this are (i) a marked increase in the startle response that does not habituate and (ii) a rise in temperature. There is no general hyper-reactivity nor somnolence. Treatment with PCPA, which prevents the synthesis of 5HT leads to complete insomnia that lasts for days. Injections of 5HT or of melatonin into the preoptic region induce sleep and injections of NE induce arousal, but excess NE also induces sleep. 5HTP plus MAOI can inhibit learning (Aprison and Hingtgen, 1965) and the time course of the disruption of behaviour correlates in time course with the rise in 5HT in the telencephalon and midbrain. Raising brain 5HT also increases SS (Poschel and Ninteman, 1968). Possibly the 5HT produced by carboxylase at the NE sites can release NE which would be the actual agent raising SS rates. Lowering levels of 5HT by reserpine or phenylalanine can potentiate learning (Stevens et al, 1967). Lesions of the MFB cause an increase in the sensitivity to electric shock. This correlates in time with the fall in brain 5HT, and the effect could be due to denervation hypersensitivity (Harvey and Lints, 1965). Emotional strains of male mice have higher brain levels of 5HT than do non-emotional strain mice.

The retina contains many 5HT neurons and a pathway leads from there to the pineal gland via the inferior accessory optic tract, the MFB and the tectum. This mediates the control of the synthesis of melatonin by the external lighting (Moore et al, 1967). Radioactive 5HTP placed in the eye is transported by these neurones and ends up around cells in the anterior and lateral hypothalamus in the region of the MFB (O'Steen and Vaughan, 1968). The functions of melatonin include inhibition of the secretion of luteinizing harmone and control of thyroid function (Fraschini et al, 1968).

Chapter 8

THEORIES OF FUNCTI

OF THE LIMBIC SYSTEM.

8.1 Early theories

The original theory of function of the limbic system—or 'rhinen-cephalon' as it was then called—was that it subserved olfaction. There is now abundant evidence that only a small portion of the amygdala and surrounding cortex has this function. In 1933 Herrick suggested that the limbic system might act as a non-specific activator of all cortical activities, influencing the internal apparatus of general bodily attitude, disposition and feeling tone. Kleist, in 1934, saw the limbic structures as basic for emotional behaviour, attitudes and drives and for correlating visceral sensations to subserve the search for food and sexual objects. Then in 1937 Papez suggested that the circuit that now bears his name was concerned with the higher elaboration of emotion.

More recently general theories of limbic function have been put forward at various degrees of elaboration. Gloor (1956) has suggested that the limbic system mediates control of functional patterns elaborated and integrated in hypothalamic and teg-mental regions by the neocortex. In particular 'One may thus conceive of this sytem (the amygdala) as more generally con-cerned with motivating reinforcement of behavioural patterns'. The basic defect produced by these lesions could then be des-cribed as a disturbance in those motivating mechanisms which normally allow the selection of behaviour appropriate to a given situation. Delgado has suggested that the specific sensory system carries information about the environment (including the state of the body), the RF is concerned with arousal and alerting functions and the limbic system with motivation. Olds (1959) in a variant of this tripartite arrangement posits that: (i) the specific sensory systems subserve selection and coding (ii) the HC–fornix–epithalamic system—learning and memory and (iii) the amygdala-hypothalamic system—motivation. Olds notes that all these three systems correlate in both directions with the three-stage reticular core (midbrain RF, thalamic RF and septal nuclei). He sees the septal nuclei as integrating higher functions of motivation and memory; the midbrain RF as integrating sensory function and in particular comparing sensory input with interpreted messages from the sensory cortex; and the thalamic RF to correlate (i) and (ii) and then as sending the final messages to the motor cortex to elicit behaviour. However, he injects a note of warning about taking speculations of this sort too seriously: 'Let the fact that the hippocampus changes function with each new experiment set the tone of tentativeness in this formulation.' Brady (1962) urges similar caution. He states that physiological studies seem to show that there is a lack of any clear-cut topographical organization for specific behavioural components but that there seems to be instead an extensive overlap in the representations within the limbic system. Olds (1958) emphasizes that the function of different anatomical areas can alter according to the circumstances. 'There are areas of the brain which are differentially affected by certain needs of the organism.' Under the influence of a particular need a given area will elicit an adaptive response aimed at the immediate repair of that need and at influencing learned responses in the direction of selecting any appropriate plan of behaviour for long-term avoidance of such needs, as far as possible, in the future. Other specific needs will evoke quite other patterns of activity if the same brain area is activated (by natural or artificial stimulation) under their influence. Delgado (1964) suggests that 'behaviour' is compounded from a mosaic of 'behavioural fragments' —each one of which is subserved by a different and specialized neuronal mechanism. These fragments are constantly being assembled and reassembled in different patterns and subpatterns for different purposes. For example 'licking' involves many muscles and ancillary systems working in a complex order and it takes part in quite different behavioural responses (e.g. alimentary, body cleaning, exploration of surroundings, maternal, etc.). In each of these recognizable much the same subpattern of behaviour is linked up as part of a different larger pattern requiring other systems (limb muscles, respiration, object selection, swallowing, etc.) to co-ordinate in an even more complex pattern. Furthermore tongue movements similar to those seen in licking take part in quite different functions (e.g. spitting, chewing, etc.). There is not one 'licking' centre (nor 'spitting', 'chewing', 'aggression', etc. centres), but in each of these activities the cortex, amygdala, hypothalamus, thalamus, RF, HC, et al are all involved. There is an interplay of dynamic and flexible patterns of neuronal excitation. Accessory brain regions such as the cerebellum and the extrapyramidal system are also involved. Other brain centres may be recruited if a connection with them had been built up by conditioned reflex formation. Each subassembly must, Delgado concludes, be under the control of a special set of cerebral structures responsible for behaviour as a whole: and the sets and subsets themselves may be arranged in some form of hierarchical fashion.

8.2 The hippocampus

The experimental work so far reviewed agrees with clinical observations that the HC is necessary for laying down a permanent memory store. In humans the memory of a recent stimulus is retained (most probably) in the primary sensory cortex as long as attention is focused on this memory (that is as long as the thalamic RF is switched over to this region in this particular context). As soon as attention is turned to something else the memory is lost if both HC have been removed. Thus the HC must mediate this function of laying down memory in a more permanent store than the temporary and attention-dependent local store in the sensory cortex.

One can picture the stream of information continually feeding into the brain from the sensory inputs as coded and already partially analysed and integrated patterns of nerve impulses (*schemata*). These schemata are then passed to other cortical areas, in part by direct corticocortical connections, in part it may be supposed via the thalamus.*

Before the mechanisms for attention, motivation and the general execution of behaviour can respond to any stimulus, its meaning must be determined. Thus the widespread cortical activity set up by an incoming S serves to analyse, compare and interpret the S in terms of the previous experience of the organism. In so far as this analysis indicates that the S is important, dangerous, possibly interesting, etc. signals will be sent to the RF to 'order' general cortical arousal (to subject the incoming schemata to a fuller analysis), or to more local cortical arousal (to subserve more local interest and attention if it is that much familiar). This may be accompanied by various behavioural reactions such as the startle reaction, or the arousal response as we have described. This activity may be a particular function of the temporal lobe, according in particular to Penfield's evidence. One can then picture the processed stream of information, having been finally marshalled in the temporal lobe (and while the RF is being activated as described), sweeping into the hippocampus and the amygdala via the extensive connections available. These schemata may then circulate around the various circuits based on the HC (and the amygdala—see the next section) i.e. the Papez circuit and the probably more important one via the subthalamus.

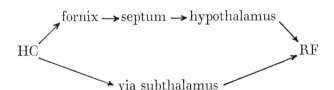

* Both the synchronization associated with external inhibition and the desynchronization associated with internal inhibition will spread to undercut motor cortex suggesting some degree of transcortical spread (John, 1961). Similarly the visual discrimination mediated by the middle and inferior temporal gyri is conducted by corticocortical paths from the striate cortex to these gyri. This learning is unaffected by lesions of the parastriate region, pulvinar nucleus or cortical undercutting of these temporal gyri: it is abolished by cortical ablation or cross-hatching.

In these circuits (and their attendant nuclei and cortical areas) close integration can be achieved between the information of the immediate state of the environment (external and internal) and the needs of the organism (because these same circuits are used extensively by the amygdala) and the appropriate schemata representing the appropriate emotional and behavioural responses can be organized in the light of this information and finally fed to motor cortex (and to the hypothalamic mechanisms of emotional and neuroendocrine activation). The unimportant schemata (those unreinforced, i.e. *those that do not lead to concomitant and appropriate amygdala function*, q.v.) die out and the important ones return (now fully integrated with the emotions that accompanied the experience) to be stored in the long-term memory stores (possibly in temporal neocortex). Adey (1965) postulates that the memory trace may be laid down elsewhere than temporal neo-cortex: 'My own notion [is] that the hippocampus is pacemaker in this respect, and that the more complex manifestations of hippo-campal rhythms that appear in the subthalamus, midbrain and visual cortex may be the physiological concomitants of both deposition and recall.' This circuit operation may explain the findings of Lesse et al (1955) reported above. It will be recalled that they stimulated the thalamic RF and recorded from the HC and obtained a dual response—a complex wave of short latency followed by a very similar one 300–500 m.sec later. The form of this second wave was drastically changed by attention. Possibly the second wave represents the packet of schemata on its return from its journey round the HC–RF circuits modified in the manner that we have suggested.

If we look again at the circuit diagram of the HC (figure 15) it would appear to constitute a mechanism for comparing two spatiotemporal patterns of neuronal excitation ('engrams'). The input from the entorhinal cortex cannot fire the HC pyramids by itself but it can preset a pattern of neurones to fire if a comple-mentary pattern is received via the input from the septum. If this happens the cells will fire and presumably send a signal to the next elements in the system that input X had such and such characteristics. If the pathway from the entorhinal cortex carries processed information from the environment and the septal input carries information from the hypothalamus about the motivational state of the organism, the HC could act as a mechanism determining what data are significant enough to put in the permanent memory store. And if the septal inflow carries information *from* the permanent memory store, the HC could function as a mechanism to classify and codify the sensory input in terms of the previous experience of the organism. Since the evidence reviewed earlier

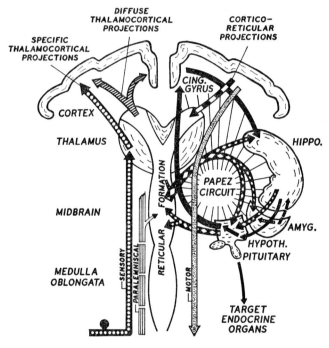

Figure 24.   Some of the limbic circuits (from H. E. Himwich)

indicates that the HC is concerned both in the laying down of permanent memories and in the correlation of the sensory input with the motivational state of the organism, it is possible that the same matching device could perform both functions in one operation. The paths from the dentate gyrus to CA 3 neurones and the Schaeffer collaterals could offer delay circuits for dealing in the same way with temporal patterns in the input, as we have suggested the HC uses to deal with spatially arrayed patterns.

The two-way traffic in most of these circuits may represent in part feedback control as well as the need for simple information flow in the other direction (e.g. hypothalamus to temporal cortex conveying information of state of internal environment) plus the complex switching and subpattern selection operations of the

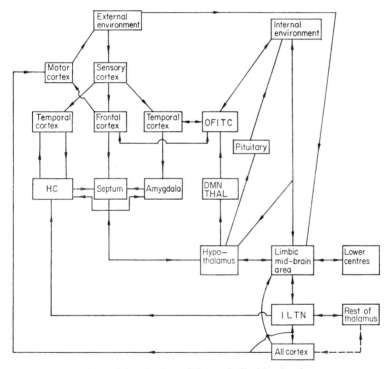

Figure 25.   A plan of the main limbic circuits

RF (cf. the important RF–hypothalamic–septal–HC circuit that we have described controlling the HC theta rhythm). The system of limbic circuits and their correlated neocortical and nuclear 'off-shoots' depicted in figures 24 and 25 cannot but remind one of the Krebs cycle. The arrangement of a circuit, or interlocking systems of circuits, whether chemical or neuroanatomical, offers many advantages for control purposes. A system where everthing is carried from cortical and subcortical areas to the RF by direct to-and-fro circuits for 'highest integration' would be expected to lead to a traffic jam at the RF.

There is some evidence to suggest that this 'inflow' does not take place via the HC gyrus. Brazier (1964) reports that the latency for an evoked potential to a flash S in the HC in man is 25–30 m.sec whereas in the HC gyrus it is 'considerably' more—which is the opposite to what one would expect. Possibly the information is fed mainly from sensory cortex to frontal cortex (possibly some via temporal cortex and the uncinate fasciculus) and enters the limbic circuits via the septal areas or by the powerful projection from the medial frontal cortex to the HC via the cingulum; another route would be by corticothalamic connections and thence to the limbic circuits; or perhaps temporal cortex outside the HC gyrus feeds directly to HC and not via this gyrus. The route via the frontal cortex is suggested by Grey Walter's discovery of the expectancy wave to which we have already referred. If the frontal lobe plays some part in the computation of the contingency of external stimuli, this route would mean that this important step in the processing of information would occur at an early stage en route to the limbic system. Sensory signals travel to the frontal cortex with very short latency and, if processed signals are there fed into the limbic circuits via the septal nuclei, this would account in part for the strategic importance of the latter and would be in line with their posited highest RF function of central switching and control.

The HC appears to have other functions besides laying down memory and acting as a way-station on the limbic circuits. It appears to have some 'switching' functions in connection with attention. In particular it appears to have a mutually inhibitory relationship with the RF in the processes of arousal and attention. Specifically it is activated by the RF in the early stages of attention, is then inhibited and finally its reactivation in turn inhibits the orientation response organized from the RF. Similarly simultaneous stimulation of the fornix and the preoptic area has been reported by Grastyán (1960), to induce forced attention (the 'sensory fixation reaction') in which the animal cannot take its eyes from a moving object. Grastyán suggests that one function of HC is to prevent an individual from diverting his attention (by its inhibitory effect on the orientation reflex).

The inhibitory function of the HC over the pituitary–adrenal stress mechanism has already been reviewed. The HC has also been reported to inhibit exploratory behaviour and to play an important role in inhibiting unwanted responses and allowing the organism to respond appropriately to novel stimuli. These functions may all be subsumed under the common function of analysing the sensory input for items of relevance in terms of the current needs and past history of the organism.

The objection might be made that the importance of these circuits here claimed is difficult to reconcile with the fact that cutting both fornices in the human seems to have little observable effect. The reply to this would be that these limbic circuits usually have multiple paths. In this instance the HC–fornix–hypothalamic pathway is insured by a massive direct HC–hypothalamic pathway. The latter runs rather diffusely through a part of the brain—the subthalamus—which most people do not have very clear ideas about, whereas none could miss the dramatic pathways of the fornix. However, the former may be functionally the more important and quite able to carry on HC and limbic circuit function in the absence of the latter. Indeed cases have been reported of the congenital absence of parts of the limbic system. Nathan and Smith (1950) have described one such case.

This brain, from a mentally and psychiatrically quite normal individual, lacked a corpus cellosum and fornix. The HC and HC gyri were much smaller than normal—whereas the amygdala, particularly the lateral nucleus, was much larger. This suggests that the amygdala can take over some HC function under conditions such as these. It is interesting to note that the mamillary bodies and hypothalamus were normal except for a possible paucity of cells in the tuber nuclei and ventromedial nucleus. Here presumably, as often happens in these congenital cases, other structures have taken over limbic circuit function.

8.3 The amygdala

There is clearly a close relationship between the amygdala and emotional behaviour, in particular with aggressive/submissive functions. It is less clear how this control is mediated. It may be by direct control of emotion or it may be by control of the basic mechanisms of conditioning such as reinforcement. The amygdala has clear-cut motor and sensory visceral connections and it exerts higher control over the hypothalamus. The latter can organize crude sequences of emotional behaviour without regard to environmental or motivational factors (sham rage, etc.). Its main function is to integrate lower sympathetic, parasympathetic and pituitary/adrenal mechanisms to give first-order sequences of emotionally based behaviour. Connections between the different hypothalamic nuclei could mediate these functions. The amygdala seems to mediate signals from cortical and other centres (indicating the state of the external environment) and from the visceral sensory inflow (indicating the state of the internal environment) and thus the data necessary for computing *needs* (e.g. 'more food', 'enough water', etc.). The match or mismatch of these two bodies of information (e.g. 'more food' with environmental information 'cupboard is bare'), appropriately modulated by more complex behavioural determinants (e.g. estimations of the social appropriateness of various actions mediated by the frontal cortex, estimations of the degree of success previously attained by behavioural sequence A in reducing specific need B, and other features of conditioned reflex formation) may in turn all influence two closely balanced mechanisms in the amygdala. These may organize and mediate opposing patterns of behaviour (e.g. 'stop/go'; 'attack/run away'; 'eat/don't eat') to include a variety of patterns of behavioural interaction with the environment centring on the basic functions of self-preservation and preservation of the species. The resultant instructions are then presumably carried from the amygdala via the limbic circuits (including RF) to the motor cortex (being modified on the way) and to the hypothalamus and from each of these to the final common path to effect the final complex sequences of behaviour (it will be recalled that emotionally determined movements do not depend on the integrity of the motor cortex).

The amygdala would thus receive an instruction, or may in part come to the decision, e.g. 'attack'. This is then recoded and reorganized in terms of the appropriate hypothalamic (and other) mechanisms to be activated, or modulated in order to execute this order. Clearly the widespread connections of the amygdala with the temporal neocortex as well as the frontal lobes, the hypothalamus, all parts of the RF and the visceral afferent system, enables it to exert these complex functions. Evidence has been presented of the ways in which the amygdala can modulate ongoing behaviour (as in the results of Delgado on stimulating the amygdala in freely moving animals). It seems also possibly of importance that it shares much of the HC limbic circuits as well as entering into some circuits more of its own: e.g.

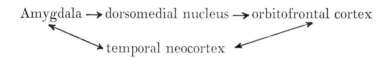

Amygdala → dorsomedial nucleus → orbitofrontal cortex
temporal neocortex

These more complex modulations from cortical regions acting both on HC and amygdala circuits or possibly on the RF directly or even on the 'final common path' may represent a third-order hierarchy of control. The neocortex is strategically placed to receive input from many parts of the limbic circuits whenever problems of greater complexity may arise needing greater computing capacity or the specialized functions located in the frontal (social analysis), parietal (spatial analysis), speech areas, etc.

The amygdala also mediates the searching response. Its role in learning appears to be subtle and complex. It may be involved in determining the reinforcement value of stimuli and with rates of extinction, also with the acquisition of CRs appropriate to situations of a higher order of complexity. Its importance in conditioned learning may be operative only until the process has been learned or overlearned. This role in computing reinforcement is in concordance with its dual afferent inflow from external and internal environments; since the process of reinforcement depends on determining which *visceral* schemata (e.g. 'food arrived') are correlated with what *external* stimuli and, in particular with what reactions to these stimuli. Thus the schemata (*a*) programming an action A that leads to reinforcement (food) B may become dominant in directing behaviour because the schemata (*a*) arrived at the amygdala in a critical relationship to the schemata (*b*) that arise from B. The timing of packets of schemata travelling around the limbic circuits and, in particular, through the amygdala, may be of importance in determining their role in conditioned reflexes. The results of these computations may be stored in the amygdala (and related cortex) in the form of altered thresholds for the eliciting of this rather than that pattern of behaviour. The information (e.g. '(*a*) was followed by (*b*) 3/4 times') may also be fed via the limbic circuits to the mesencephalic and thalamic RF that are responsible for alerting, attention, control of certain features of sensory input and motor tone, etc. so that these functions are modified in the appropriate manner to deal with the situation (e.g. how best to deal with S when, previously (when S) then (*a*) → (*b*) 3/4 times).

The amygdala is a moderately powerful centre for reward and punishment (using Olds's technique) and it exerts powerful control over the pituitary/adrenal function in an opposite direction to that exerted by the HC. Wurtz and Olds (1963) see the amygdala in this role: 'It is generally agreed that the amygdaloid complex is a correlative or modulating structure within the brain's system of motivating and emotional mechanisms.' In amygdala lesions there may be interference with environmental control over the organism. In hypothalamic lesions in contrast there is loss of motivational control of behaviour by the physiological state of the organism (e.g. the animal does not stop eating when satiated or does not eat when hungry). There is also some evidence that the amygdala mediates a rapid 'alarm' system. The specific 45 c/s rhythm is set off by significant or dangerous system and the amygdala can rapidly activate the pituitary/adrenal stress mechanism.

Thus, to put the matter crudely, the HC may lay down

memories, the amygdala (with HC) may determine what memories are to be laid down, and the RF may subserve the complex switching and general programme organization such a complex operation requires. The entire limbic system may function to select the appropriate behaviour to any given set of stimuli. The cortex may in this context be regarded as specialized computing subsystems to deal with problems of a higher order of complexity than the subcortical nuclei can manage as well as supplying a

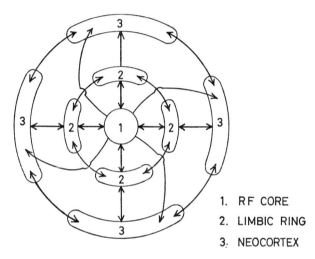

1. RF CORE
2. LIMBIC RING
3. NEOCORTEX

Figure 26. The basic forebrain plan

permanent memory store and specialized functions related to social and spatial analysis, language, etc. as has already been suggested.

Figure 26 illustrates these features of brain design. The central RF core is surrounded by the limbic circuits and these in turn by the cortical mantle. The outer layers deal with factors of increasing complexity, the inner layers with the integration of more factors. The central organizer of this system would appear to be the RF.

Delgado (1967) has extended his investigations of the effect of brain stimulation on free behaviour of monkeys living in a permanent colony. Stimulation of the anterior hypothalamus in two

L

monkeys led to a complex and specific sequence of behaviour. The monkey walked to the opposite wall, climbed up it and vocalized. The lateral hypothalamus gave only pupillary constriction and minor behavioural manifestations. The posterior hypothalamus in one monkey gave a different behavioural response—turning round, touching the wall and looking through a tube. The fimbria gave in three monkeys the same response—running rapidly round the cage but no aggressive reactions. The basolateral amygdala (two monkeys) gave a crouching reaction and behavioural inhibition. It also increased sleeping time in inter-trial periods. Delgado hypothesizes that the stimulated areas are not directly responsible for the behavioural response but they organize spatiotemporal sequences of behaviour, e.g. walking has

'. . . an anatomical and functional set represented in the motor cortex, cerebellum, basal ganglia and other structures which may be triggered for different purposes from several areas of the brain related to food intake, curiosity, nocioception, etc. . . . We could conceive of the limbic system as organizing centres which modulate the functions of other cerebral structures. The triggering area should be more directly responsible for the *behavioral sequence* and perhaps for the *purpose* of the sequence than for the motor performance. Isolated acts like flapping the ears can be evoked from a variety of cerebral locations, while *sequences of behaviour seem to be specific of determined structures*. . . . The stimulated region cannot be accepted as a "center" with determined motor outputs, but as a planning station which activates a variety of substations and organizes their functions in space and in time according to determined sequences, processing at the same time sensory information which interplays with the organization of the response'.

MacKay (1966) has postulated that the cortex is the *organizational system* of the brain that elaborates all the elaborate feedforward necessary to keep the pattern of action matched to current sensory data in obedience to normative signals from the metaorganizational system. The cortex also feeds the latter with condensed indications of cortical activity, including categorized representations of the state of the external world. The limbic system constitutes the *meta-organizational system*. This appraises and evaluates the activities of the first system and balances current priorities with regard to the short-term and long-term needs of the organism, and the selection and evaluation of different integrative activities.

Chapter 9

SOME PSYCHIATRIC

SPECULATIONS

One may wonder if any of this recently acquired body of knowledge, or these new theories of limbic function, can throw any light on clinical problems in psychiatry. Whatever view we take of the cause of psychiatric disorders it cannot be denied that explanations of them in terms of psychodynamics, or environmental factors, or generalized biochemical disorders, can be complemented and extended by descriptions of the actual brain events that occur during the on-going disordered experience or behaviour. Causation in psychiatric illness is usually multiple. A person inherits the nexus of his personality structure and biochemical idiosyncrasies. The details of his early upbringing modulate this potentiality and determine to which subsequent life stresses he will be vulnerable. The third factor is the contingent fact whether he actually is subjected to these stresses, to what degree and how he, his family and friends and his medical advisers react to them.

Let us take as an example the psychiatric illness or syndrome called depression. There appears to be a genetic factor that predisposes people to fall victim to certain types of depression—particularly the endogenous form. Secondly disorders of upbringing such as parental deprivation at critical ages act as further predisposing factors or part causes. Thirdly some psychic trauma such as the immediate loss of a loved figure may actually precipitate the attack of depression. A faulty mother–child relationship may, for example, induce in the child difficulties in forming proper human relationships in later life. The dependency needs were not resolved as they normally should be by the mother and are transferred to other people—e.g. the wife—with usually a deleterious effect on this relationship and this situation may lead eventually to a reactive depression. Many such part causes of depression may most usefully be understood in psychological, social and indeed common-sense terms. Most mild depressions get better by themselves in time because the person takes simple measures to throw off his depression (Dr Johnson would walk the 32 miles from Lichfield to Birmingham and back in search of relief of his melancholia); because psychological ego defences and physiological mechanisms of homeostasis come into play to restore normality; and because the mere passage of time tends to dilute the physiological engrams mediating the psychic trauma (bereavement, etc.) that set off the depression. In other cases of depression, however—the so-called endogenous group—the genetic factors seem to be much stronger, the previous personality is often normal, and the quality of the depression is different. It is in this group particularly that delusions occur. These are the false beliefs that the patient is wicked, deserves all manner of savage punishment, or is consumed by some loathsome disease, or is ruined, rotting away, dying. In these cases a disorder of brain physiology would seem to be the primary cause and we now have some evidence that this is concerned with the metabolism in the brain of the biogenic amines, serotonin and noradrenaline.

When a depression reaches a certain level of intensity, or has a severe disturbance of brain physiology as its main cause, various vicious circles seem to develop. The patient seems no longer able to take the ordinary measures by which mild depressions are fought (i.e. forcing oneself into activity instead of sitting around moping, forcing oneself into company instead of feeling sorry for oneself in solitude, and so on). In these cases the patient appears to be overwhelmed by the depression in spite of his excellent personality and a courageous struggle against it. Social effectiveness breaks down with much resulting secondary distress to the patient who feels irrational yet agonizing guilt at having let down his family and friends. The actions to which he is now driven—weeping, indecision, importunity, delusion formation and action arising from these, are very likely to lead to negative reactions in his family and associates which further aggravate his depression. Concomitant with these psychological and social vicious circles there may be a physiological one whereby the mechanisms of cerebral amine metabolism that are the cerebral correlate of mood may enter a stage of runaway disorder—of positive feedback—and this may be aggravated by the failure of compensatory metabolic mechanisms. Serotonin and noradrenaline are concentrated particularly in the limbic system and it is reasonable to suppose that the physiological disturbance underlying a depressive illness may have its maximum effect in this system.

The first evidence for the role of particular limbic structures in maintaining psychiatric symptoms came from the operation of prefrontal leucotomy. Cases where emotional tension, anxiety and depression are marked and intractable are often greatly helped by cutting the connections between the dorsomedial nucleus of the thalamus and the orbitofrontal cortex. It is possible that the elaboration of reactions of stress, anxiety and depression is conducted by these circuits which would be responsible for setting the thresholds and degree of generalization of these emotional reactions. An idea of how this might be done is suggested by the work of Grey Walter on the expectancy wave to which we have already referred. It will be recalled that this wave is a function of the contingency of relationship between one stimulus and another. Patients with anxiety states apparently form very strong expectancy waves (Grey Walter—personal communication). The main feature of an anxiety state is that the patient becomes anxious or even panic-stricken in response to stimuli that do not upset most people (e.g. going out of the house, meeting strangers, etc.). Complex factors of personality structure, previous conditioning and the vagaries of experience have combined in setting the thresholds of the 'fear' response too low and its level of generalization too wide and the disorder of these mechanisms can be detected electrophysiologically in terms of the disordered expectancy wave. This whole field promises to be a rewarding and rapidly expanding locus for research in neuropsychiatry and neuropsychology—in what the Russians would call 'higher brain function'.

The occurrence of depressive delusions seems to be related to the 'physiological' stage of depression. It is probable that these delusions are generated by the disordered brain mechanisms. The quality of delusion seems such that a simple psychological explanation along the lines that the patient is feeling so wretched that he comes to believe the worst is inadequate: in any case it is hardly an *explanation* for his delusion except at the rather obvious level that there is a causal link between his depressed affect and the delusions. If we look for a neurological explanation we could suggest something along the following lines. We have supposed that the great limbic circuits form the means of evaluating and integrating experience, and finally laying down what is important in the permanent memory store and discarding the dross. The amygdala seems concerned mainly with the emotional and motivational aspect of this control system and the hippocampus with the actual laying down of memory. Both are concerned with environmental factors. Thus, if the physiological malfunction of depression originates, or has its main focus, in the amygdala or hypothalamus, these may send 'depression-laden' abnormal schemata around the meta-organizational system in which the hippocampal circuits are inseparably entwined, and this may automatically engender therein the schemata that are the cerebral basis for the beliefs that the patient is wicked, ruined, dying, etc. In other words the anatomical substrate for the close link between affect and belief may be in part the fact that the amygdala and the hippocampus share the great limbic circuits, that these circuits are responsible for blending affect and ideation into a conjoined programme for behaviour. Major upsets in the emotional system impose schemata on the ideational system that represent the kind of events that might have been expected to cause, in the normal course of events, feelings of despair and dejection. Minor upsets in the emotional system do not, as it were, spill over into the ideational system but once the threshold for overspill is reached delusions and the vicious circle of depression that these delusions engender, develop. That is to say a natural reinforcement occurs between the primary physiological upset and the psychological consequences of the symptoms thereby occasioned and this can at times proceed beyond the point at which homeostatic mechanism can intervene to redress the balance.

The relationship between symptoms and physiology are of

course more complex than depicted in this simple scheme. The influence of cultural factors and learning are of great importance in determining the course and form of mental illness. The symptoms in depression of feelings of guilt and delusions of unworthiness, poverty, etc. are typical of Western cultures of the WASP (white anglo-saxon protestant) type and similar cultures, such as the Jewish, that lay great emphasis on *individual* responsibility. These symptoms are scarcely seen in other cultures, such as the southern Italian where much less stress is laid on the importance of self-reliance and the attitude is not held that personal misfortune must be the person's own fault. It is part of the great American cultural myth that anyone can succeed by hard work, good sense, thrift, etc. The reverse of the medal is the belief that failure is due to weakness, laziness, infirmity of moral character, etc. In these cultures depression leads to delusions that what is feared has actually come to pass, i.e. that the person *is* weak, wicked, etc. In other cultures misfortune is accounted for on other grounds, and much less emphasis is placed on the sturdy protestant virtues. In these cultures misfortune tends to be accounted for in terms of the evil or magical machinations of others and it is dealt with by vendetta or counter-magic. In these cultures depression as we know it is virtually unknown and the common forms of psychosis are episodes of confused excitement. Thus depression can hardly be described as an *illness* with *symptoms* of guilt, self-blame, etc.; for these symptoms vary as the cultures vary and must therefore be learned. What *does* seem to happen is that the illness leads to beliefs that *that* has happened which would in that culture have been the sort of event most likely to lead to agonizing feelings of failure, guilt, shame, etc. The mechanisms that normally couple affect to experience seem to be working in reverse so that the affects determine the ideation rather than vice-versa.

Similar considerations can be raised with respect to certain fundamental postulates of Freudian psychopathology. It will be recalled that Freud supposed that many neurotic symptoms arose from unacceptable and repressed wishes, usually of a sexual nature. Thus he supposed that there was a causal link between aberrant sexual development *per se* and neurosis. However it seems likely that cultural factors complicate this account. Freudian psychology was developed in nineteenth-century Vienna, in a Victorian culture in which sex was taboo and a vehicle for the maximum shame and embarrassment. Hence the culture determined what was unacceptable to consciousness. In a sexually permissive culture guilt and shame would not be conditioned to sexual matters and the latter would not be expected to play a prominent part in the genesis of neurosis. Neurosis can be regarded as a function of conditioning. In any culture, fear, guilt, shame are conditioned to certain acts, events, attitudes, and so on. This often entails the control of instinctual drives within limits determined by the culture. Animal experimentation has abundantly shown that syndromes very like human neurosis can be developed by conflict situations of various kinds. The failure to resolve two powerful behavioural programmes competing for dominance tends to neurosis, whether the conflict is due to a constant presentation of stimuli with ambiguous threat/reward meaning, or whether it is due to the need to suppress behaviour (or even the desire for such behaviour) that is unacceptable to the culture.

For example the Indians of Ontario used to live in fear of starvation in the long, hard winters and they might be expected to entertain unacceptable ideas of being forced into cannibalism in order to survive. These people exhibit a form of psychosis—the Wittigo psychosis—where the delusions develop that the person has become a cannibal; that is, the belief developed that that which is most feared by the culture has come to pass.

It seems unlikely that repressed homosexual desires (the cause posited by Freud for so much neurosis in our culture) would have operated in cultures such as the fourth century B.C. Theban culture where homosexuality was regarded as quite normal and thus homosexual desires did not have to be repressed.

If we are to look for a physiological basis for neurosis certain avenues suggest themselves: for example, the mechanisms of conflict of behavioural patterns, and the learning of socially required control of aggression and other instinctual drives. If the limbic circuits provide the mechanism for laying down of memory, it is reasonable to suppose that they are also concerned with active forgetting—i.e. repression. The role of the hippocampus in this is suggested by the experiments of Webster and Voneida (1964) quoted on page 72. The physiological basis for the undesirable effects of 'repression' may be the fact that painful memories, no longer available to the mechanisms of conscious recall, may nevertheless be available to the neurologically somewhat distinct mechanisms of emotional control and may play havoc in the hypothalamus, pre-motor cortex, etc. leading to symptoms such as depression, anxiety and hysterical paralysis. Other neurotic symptoms may not derive from repression but from faulty conditioning of the delicate mechanisms responsible for the control of emotion and behaviour. Indeed it would be remarkable if so complex a mechanism possessed only one major manner of breakdown. Chronic fear, anxiety, terror, depression themselves may well cause secondary disruptions in other brain functions such as attention, speech, sleep, feeding. The occurrence of disturbances of sleep, of appetite, of libido, of the powers of attention and concentration in neurosis suggests that a disturbance of one aspect of limbic function (anxiety, depression, etc.) induces a disorder in other limbic functions. This suggests (i) that the underlying biochemical lesion upsets a mechanism involved in all these limbic functions and/or (ii) that a disturbance of one limbic function necessarily involves an upset in other limbic function. If the function of the limbic system is the close integration of many disparate brain functions into one orderly whole, then the penalty for this may be the inability of such a system to localize a disturbance in one of its subsystems to that subsystem. The price of integration may be multiplicity of symptoms in neurosis.

A second important factor in neurosis, emphasized by Freud, is the importance of infantile sexuality. If we look at this idea in a cultural and ethological framework we can note the importance of the first experience of any organism for its subsequent patterns of behaviour as disclosed in the ethological study of imprinting. But we can go on to suggest that it, and not disorders in development of infantile sexuality *per se*, is the causal agent in neurosis. It may be of more importance that in our culture evidences of sexuality before the culturally approved age, toilet training, etc. are often the *first* occasion when scandalized punishment is inflicted on the child; that is when shame and guilt are imprinted. Similarly the absence of a mother- or father-figure at certain critical ages seems to induce a failure of the development of the mechanisms responsible for the long-term direction of behaviour due in part to a disorder of imprinting and complex conditioning, that lead to life-long inabilities in forming adequate interpersonal relationships. The severe disruption of the ability to adopt adequate social control and to form these social relationships that follow on the old standard leucotomy suggests that the lateral surface of the frontal lobe has a significant part to play in this social control. This part of the cortex seems specialized to deal with the evaluation and elaboration of behavioural patterns in which complex social factors are involved: just as the parietal lobe seems to deal with the analysis of complex spatial factors in sensorimotor function.

In the case of the neuroses the disturbances of brain function seem to remain localized to limbic functions. No severe language disturbances occur, no thought disorder, no disturbance of parietal, temporal or frontal lobe function. Schizophrenia, on the other hand, seems to be marked by a *wider* disturbance of brain function to include much of the temporal lobe (the hallucinations and the many disorders in the evaluation of experience typical of aberrant temporal lobe function) together with a severe disruption of functions in which the limbic system plays an important part, e.g. emotion, thinking and the relationship between them. It is well known that cases of temporal lobe epilepsy can develop a psychosis indistinguishable from schizophrenia due apparently simply to chronic malfunction of the temporal lobe. We have noted that other mental disorders seem to be characterized by a basic emotion getting into a state of runaway disequilibrium (e.g. the anxiety state (fear), depression (melancholy), mania (elation)). In schizophrenia the emotional complexes that could play a similar role would seem to be those with a *necessary* interpersonal factor—such as the suspicion, submissiveness, malignant shyness etc. of the schizoid personality. However, the simple model of an emotion entering a phase of 'positive feedback' does not do justice to the complex clinical features of schizophrenia. In this disease it is possible that there is a disturbance of brain physiology (Smythies, 1963) and there may also be disturbances of limbic and temporal lobe function brought about by learning and the social stigma of having an unmentionable disease. Cultural features are important in schizophrenia. It is possibly significant that the delusions of schizophrenia are totally unacceptable to our culture. The delusions of endogeneous depression are all in terms of ruin, guilt and sickness that is readily understandable in our culture. The delusions of schizophrenia tend to be in terms of witchcraft, telepathy, possession, communion with God, etc. that lead to immediate exclusion and rejection by the culture. Possibly the malignancy of schizophrenia reflects this total cultural rejection. In other cultures that believe in witchcraft, possession, spirits, etc. naturally such beliefs are not regarded as 'delusions' but as ordinary attitudes for which the culture is perfectly prepared and for which there are rules by which to deal with them. In certain Siberian tribes, for example, people who have what in our eyes would be regarded as undoubted and alarming acute schizophrenic breakdowns become leaders of society—the Shamans. The 'hallucinatory' experiences and the 'deluded' beliefs are regarded as perfectly normal instances of communication with the all-important spirit world and as necessary training for someone who would wish to become a leader of that society with the leader's responsibility for protecting the tribe from evil spirits.

To conclude therefore we can postulate the following:

1. The neuroses represent quantitative disturbances of limbic control of the emotions and behaviour where the faulty patterns of feeling and behaviour are determined very largely by faulty conditioning and faulty setting of thresholds and generalizations in the way that we have described. There is no change in the normal ideation → emotion causal chain and no qualitative change in brain physiology.

2. In the psychoses there seem to be qualitative changes in brain physiology. Or rather that the quantitative changes in such systems as serotonin, noradrenaline and dopamine metabolism or the biochemical processes of methylation become so

serious that homeostasis breaks down and the various vicious circles that we have described develop. The causal chain ideation → emotion reverses. In depression the disorder may be limited to the limbic system and in schizophrenia a more widespread disorder of brain function may be involved including the temporal lobe. This wider spread may occur for several reasons. The basic biochemical lesion, if there is such, may affect more widespread mechanisms. The emotions that become disordered may cause more widespread havoc. The delusions and behaviour manifest in the disease may result in greater cultural rejection, with consequent intensification of feelings of insecurity, rejection, suspicion, hatred, etc.

In the present state of our knowledge of brain function these speculations are necessarily sketchy. They are merely meant to illustrate the kind of conceptual framework we could use in order to give an account of the origins of mental illness in all its complexity in physiological language. Such an endeavour is complementary to the extensive applications of learning theory that have been made to symptom formation that lie outside the scope of this review. Nevertheless our knowledge of the *actual processes* by which the brain organizes emotion, thinking and behaviour is daily increasing. When these actual processes are known the need for employing interim models such as is contained in much of Freudian psychopathology becomes progressively less useful. The neurologist Freud was forced to adopt a dualistic model in the 1890s in the absence of any information about higher brain function. However, he recognized the interim nature of his psychopathology and that eventually the translation of his explanations of human behaviour into physiological terms must take place. This step is made inevitable by the nature of scientific explanation itself. Science progresses in many ways, but scientists of all persuasions are agreed that one important way is to develop and extend explanations given at one level of the hierarchy of science in terms of the theories and concepts of the science one higher in the hierarchy. Chemistry can give a very useful account of phenomena in terms of interactions at the atomic and molecular level. In this account a great number of statements about events must be accepted as basic statements that can be used to explain phenomena but cannot themselves be so explained within the system. For example chemistry explains the interaction between hydrogen and chlorine in terms of the valency theory. But the fact that hydrogen has a valency of 1 is simply a basic fact in the system and we cannot answer the question 'Why has hydrogen a valency of 1?' within the concepts of the system. In order to do so we have to move up to the next step of the hierarchy to atomic physics where explanations are available in terms of electron shells, etc. that enable us to answer this question. Similarly Freudian psychopathology cannot really answer the question 'But why should repressed wishes lead to such symptoms' except in terms of an *analogy* with the flow of physical energy. Such a model is descriptive rather than explanatory; or rather its explanatory power depends on the contingent accident of the degree of similarity that there happens to be between the operation of the complex brain mechanisms that actually organize psychic life and behaviour on the one hand and the properties of the kind of physical energy, e.g. electric currents, that were familiar to Freud in 1890 and on which he based his model.

Physiology, in turn, is developed in terms of chemistry, and psychology in turn in terms of neurophysiology, cybernetics and neurochemistry, etc. That is not to say that any part of Freudian or any other system of psychology or psychopathology is necessarily *wrong*. It is merely that they are likely to become superseded by more powerful systems of explanation in terms of what actually goes on in the brain when people behave normally or aberrantly. The test of any such development is whether it can account for separate elements of the earlier system by showing that they all necessarily follow from explanations given in the more advanced system. The more advanced system can trace causal connections between events that the earlier system had to accept as merely contingent companions. For example psychiatry to date has accepted the occurrence of delusions in depression on a contingent basis as merely a symptom among other symptoms, much as spots in measles were merely a symptom of measles before anything was known about viruses and how the spots were actually caused. We have put forward the hypothesis that delusions occur in depression because the amygdala and the hippocampus share the same neurological circuits; that these circuits serve to co-ordinate affect with experience and ideation; that normally the causal chain operates in the direction experience and ideation → affect; and that in depression this causal chain reverses to produce delusions (and even hallucinations if experience is affected as well as ideation). This hypothesis is very crude and may of course be quite wrong. But it is the kind of hypothesis that is required.*

The experimental and conceptual ground-work for this development is at present being laid and its brave if rather sketchy beginnings are reviewed in this book.

* Such hypotheses may eventually be tested by experiment.

References

Adey, W.R. (1959) *Int. Rev. Neurobiol.*, **1**, 1.

Adey, W.R. (1965) Personal Communication.

Adey, W.R. (1967) *Prog. Brain Res.*, **27**, 228.

Adey, W.R., Merrilees, N.C.R. and Sunderland, S. (1956) *Brain*, **79**, 414.

Adey, W.R., Walter, D.O. and Lindsey, D.F. (1962) *Arch. Neurol.*, **6**, 194.

Akert, K., Gruesson, R.A., Woolsey, C.N. and Meyer, D.R. (1961) *Brain*, **84**, 480.

Allen, W.F. (1938) *Amer. J. Physiol.*, **121**, 657.

Allen, W.F. (1940) *Amer. J. Physiol.*, **128**, 754.

Allikinets, L.H. and Lapin, I.P. (1967) *Int. J. Neuropharm.*, **6**, 99.

Altman, J. (1967) in *The Neurosciences* (G. C. Quarton, T. Melnechuk and F. O. Schmitt, eds.), New York, Rockefeller University Press.

Anand, B.K. and Brobeck, J.R. (1951) *Yale J. Biol. Med.*, **24**, 123.

Anderson, B., Gale, C.C., Hökfelt, B. and Larsson, B. (1965) *Acta Physiol. Scand.*, **65**, 45.

Anderson, P., Holmqvist, B. and Voorhoeve, P.E. (1966) *Acta Physiol. Scand.*, **66**, 461.

Aprison, M.H. and Hingtgen, J.N. (1965) *J. Neurochem.*, **12**, 959.

Bagshaw, M.H. and Benzies, S. (1968) *Exp. Neurol.*, **20**, 175.

Bagshaw, M.H. and Coppock, H.W. (1968) *Exp. Neurol.*, **20**, 188.

Baile, C.A., Scott, F.A. and Mayer, J. (1967) *Experentia*, **23**, 1033.

Baird, H.N., Gudetti, B., Reyes, V., Wycis, H.T. and Spiegel, E.G. (1951) *Fed. Proc.*, **10**, 8.

Baker, W.W. and Benedict, F. (1968) *Int. J. Neuropharm.*, **7**, 135.

Barbizet, J. (1963) *J. Neurol. Neurosurg. Psychiat.* **26**, 127.

Bard, P. and Mountcastle, V.B. (1948) 'Some forebrain mechanisms involved in expression of rage with special reference to suppression of angry behavior' in *The Frontal Lobe* (J. Fulton, ed.), Williams & Wilkins, Baltimore, 362–404.

Barker, D.J. (1967) *J. comp. physiol. Psychol.*, **64**, 453.

Barondes, S.H. and Cohen, H.D. (1968) *Science*, **160**, 556.

Bar-Sela, M.E. and Critchelow, V. (1966) *Amer. J. Physiol.*, **211**, 1103.

Biscoe, T.J. and Straughan, D.W. (1966) *J. Physiol.*, **183**, 341.

Bizzi, E., Malliani, A., Apelbaum, J. and Zanchetti, A. (1963) *Arch. Ital. Biol.*, **101**, 614.

Bleier, R., Bard, P. and Woods, J.W. (1966) *J. comp. Neurol.*, **128**, 255.

Bohus, B. (1961) *Acta Physiol. Acad. Sci. Hung.*, **20**, 373.

Bohus, B. and de Wied, D. (1967) *J. comp. physiol. Psychol.*, **64**, 26.

Bond, D.D., Randt, C.T., Bidder, T.G. and Rowland, V. (1957) *Arch. Neurol. Psychiat.*, **78**, 143.

Brady, J.V. (1958) 'The paleocortex and behavioral motivation' in *Biological* and *Biochemical Basis of Behavior* (H. F. Harlow and C. N. Woolsey, eds.). Madison, University of Wisconsin Press, pp. 193–235.

Brady, J.V. (1962) 'Psychophysiology of emotional behavior' in *Experimental Foundations of Clinical Psychology* (A. J. Bachrach, ed.), Basic Books.

Brady, J.V. and Conrad, D.G. (1960) *J. exp. anal. Behav.*, **3**, 93.

Brazier, M.A.B. (1964) *Ann. N.Y. Acad. Sci.*, **112**, 33.

Bremner, F.J. (1964) *J. comp. physiol. Psychol.*, **58**, 16.

Bromiley, R.B. (1948) *J. comp. physiol. Psychol.*, **41**, 102.

Brown, B.B. (1968) *EEG clin. Neurophysiol.*, **24**, 53.

Brown, S. and Schaeffer, E.A. (1888) *Phil. Trans. Roy. Soc. London*, **179B**, 303.

Brutowski, S., Fonberg, E. and Mempel, E. (1960) *Acta biol. Exp.*, **20**, 263.

Buchwald, N.A. and Ervin, F.R. (1957) *EEG clin. Neurophysiol.*, **9**, 477.

Burešová, O. and Bureš, J. (1965) *Acta Physiol. Acad. Sci. Hung.*, **26**, 53.

Burešová, O., Bureš, J., Fifkova, E., Vinogradova, O. and Weiss, T. (1962) *Exp. Neurol.*, **6**, 161.

Burkett, E.E. and Bunnell, B.N. (1966) *J. comp. physiol. Psychol.*, **62**, 468.

Carey, J.H. (1957) *J. comp. Neurol.*, **108**, 57.

Chance, M. and Silverman, P. (1964) *Proc. 3rd Congress. Colleg. Internat. Neuropsychopharmacologicum.* Birmingham.

Chase, M.H., Sterman, M.B. and Clemente, C.D. (1966) *Exp. Neurol.*, **16**, 36.

Chatrian, G.E. and Chapman, W.R. (1960) 'Electrographic studies of the amygdaloid region with implanted electrodes in patients with temporal lobe epilepsy' in *Electrical Studies on the Unanaesthetized brain*. (E. R. Ramey and D. S. O'Doherty, eds.), Hoeber, New York.

Chow, K.L. (1961) 'Anatomical and electrographic analysis in temporal neocortex in relation to visual discrimination learning in monkeys' in *Brain Mechanisms and Learning* (J. F. Delafresnaye, ed.), Oxford, Blackwell Scientific Publications, p. 507.

Clark, C.V.H. and Isaacson, R.L. (1965) *J. comp. physiol. Psychol.*, **59**, 137.

Coons, E.E., Lewak, M. and Miller, N.E. (1965) *Science*, **150**, 1320.

Correll, R.E. (1957) *J. comp. physiol. Psychol.*, **50**, 624.

Correll, R.E. and Scoville, W. (1965) *J. comp. physiol. Psychol.*, **60**, 360.

Cowan, W.M., Raisman, G. and Powell, T.P.S. (1965) *J. Neurol. Neurosurg. Psychiat.*, **28**, 137.

Dahl, D., Ingram, W.R. and Knott, J.R. (1962) *Arch. Neurol.*, **7**, 314.

Delgado, J.M.R. (1964) *Int. Rev. Neurobiol.*, **6**, 349.

Delgado, J.M.R. (1967) *Prog. Brain Res.*, **27**, 48.

Deutsch, J.A. (1962) *Ann. Rev. Physiol.*, **24**, 259.

Deutsch, J.A. and Lutsky, H. (1967) *Nature*, **213**, 742.

Deutsch, J.A. and Rocklin, K.W. (1967) *Nature*, **216**, 89.

de Wied, D. (1965) *Int. J. Neuropharmacol.*, **4**, 157.

Diamond, M.C., Krech, D. and Rosenzweig, M.R. (1964) *J. comp. Neurol.*, **123**, 111.

M

Dicara, L.V. and Wolf, G. (1968) *Exp. Neurol.*, **21**, 231.

Domino, E.F. (1968) *EEG clin. Neurophysiol.*, **24**, 292.

Domino, E.F. and Olds, M.E. (1968) *J. Pharm. exp. Therap.*, **164**, 202.

Donovan, B.T. (1966) *Brit. Med. Bull.*, **22**, 249.

Douglas, R.J. (1967) *Psych. Bull.*, **67**, 416.

Douglas, R.J. and Raphelson, A.C. (1966) *J. comp. physiol. Psychol.*, **62**, 320 and 465.

Drachman, D.A. and Ommaya, A.K. (1964) *Arch. Neurol.*, **10**, 411.

Drachman, D.A. and Arbit, J. (1966) *Arch. Neurol.*, **15**, 52.

Dreifuss, J.J. and Murphy, J.T. (1968) *Brain Res.*, **8**, 167.

Dunlop, C.W. (1958) *EEG clin. Neurophysiol.*, **10**, 297.

Egger, M.D. and Flynn, J.P. (1963) *J. Neurophysiol.*, **26**, 705.

Ehrlich, A. (1964) *Psych. Bull.*, **61**, 100.

Elazar, Z. and Adey, W.R. (1967) *Prog. Brain Res.*, **27**, 218.

Eleftheriou, E. and Boehlke, K.W. (1967) *Science*, **155**, 1693.

Ellen, P. and Powell, E.W. (1962) *Exp. Neurol.*, **6**, 538.

Ellen, P. and Powell, E.W. (1963) *Science*, **141**, 828.

Ellen, P. and Powell, E.W. (1966) *Exp. Neurol.*, **16**, 162.

Ellen, P., Wilson, A.S. and Powell, E.W. (1964) *Exp. Neurol.*, **10**, 120.

Elliott Smith, G. (1910) *Lancet*, **i**, 147 and 221.

Elul, R. (1964) *EEG Clin. Neurophysiol.*, **16**, 489.

Endröczi, E. and Lissák, K. (1962) *Acta Physiol. Acad. Sci. Hung.*, **22**, 265.

Endröczi, E., Lissák, K., Bohus, B. and Kovacs, S. (1959) *Acta Physiol. Acad. Sci. Hung.*, **16**, 17.

Feldberg, W., Hellon, R.F. and Lotti, V.J. (1967) *J. Physiol.*, **191**, 501.

Feldman, S. (1962) *Exp. Neurol.*, **5**, 269.

Fendler, K., Karmos, G., and Telegdy, G. (1961) *Acta Physiol. Acad. Sci. Hung.*, **20**, 293.

Fernadez De Molina, A. and Hunsperger, R.W. (1962) *J. Physiol.*, **160**, 200.

Folkow, B., and Rubenstein, E. H. (1966) *Acta Physiol. Scan.*, **66**, 182.

Fonberg, E. (1963) *Acta biol. Exp.*, **23**, 171.

Fraschini, F., Mess, B., Pira, F. and Martini, L. (1968) *Science*, **159**, 1104.

Freeman, W.J. (1963) *Int. Rev. Neurobiol.*, **5**, 53.

Fuller, J.L., Rosvold, H.E. and Pribram, K.H. (1957) *J. comp. physiol. Psychol.*, **50**, 89.

Fuxe, K., Hamberger, B. and Hökfelt, T. (1968) *Brain Res.*, **8**, 125.

Galambos, R. (1961) 'Changing concepts of the learning mechanism' in *Brain Mechanisms and Learning* (J. F. Delafresnaye, ed.), Oxford, Blackwell Scientific Publications, pp. 231–41.

Gastaut, H. (1958) 'Some aspects of the neurophysiological basis of conditioned reflexes and behaviour' in *The Neurological Basis of Behaviour*. Ciba Foundation Symposium (G. E. W. Wolstenholme and C. M. O'Connor, eds.), Churchill, London, pp. 255–72.

Gergen, J.A. and Maclean, P.D. (1964) *Ann. N.Y. Acad. Sci.*, **117**, 69.

Gloor, P. (1956) 'Telencephalic influences upon the hypothalamus' in *Hypothalamic–Hypophyseal Interrelationships* (W. S. Fields, ed.), C. C. Thomas, Springfield, 74–113.

Gloor, P., Sperti, L. and Vera, C.L. (1963) *EEG Clin. Neurophysiol.*, **15**, 353.

Goddard, G.V. (1964) *J. comp. physiol. Psych.*, **58**, 23.

Grant, L.D. and Jarrard, L.E. (1968) *Brain Res.*, **10**, 392.

Grastyán, E. (1959) in *The Central Nervous System and Behavior* (M. A. B. Brazier, ed.), Trans. 2nd Conf. Josiah Macy Jr. Foundation, Madison, Madison Printing Co.

Grastyán, E. (1961) 'The significance of the earliest manifestation of conditioning in the mechanism of learning' in *Brain Mechanisms and Learning* (J. F. Delafresnaye, ed.), Oxford, Blackwell Scientific Publications, p. 243.

Grastyán, E., Karmos, G., Vereczkey, L. and Kellenyi, E.E. (1966) *EEG clin. Neurophysiol.*, **21**, 34.

Green, J.D. (1958a) 'The rhinencephalon and behaviour' in *The Neurological Basis of Behaviour*, Ciba Foundation Symposium (G. E. W. Wolstenholme and C. M. O'Connor, eds.), London, Churchill.

Green, J.D. (1958b) 'The rhinencephalon: aspects of its relation to behaviour and the reticular activating system' in *Reticular Formation of the Brain* (H. H. Jasper et al, eds.), London, Churchill.

Green, J.D. (1964) *Physiol. Rev.*, **44**, 561.

Green, J.D., Clemente, C.D. and de Groot, J. (1967a) *J. comp. Neurol.*, **108**, 505.

Green, J.D., Clemente, C.D. and de Groot, J. (1967b) *Arch. Neurol. Psychiat.*, **78**, 259.

Green, J.D., Duisberg, R.E.H. and McGrath, W.B. (1951) *J. Neurosurg.*, **8**, 157.

Gregory, R. (1961) 'The brain as an engineering problem' in *Current Problems in Animal Behaviour* (W.H. Thorpe and O.L. Zangwill, eds.), Cambridge University Press.

Grossman, S.P. (1964a) *J. comp. physiol. Psych.*, **57**, 29.

Grossman, S.P. (1964b) *J. comp. physiol. Psych.*, **58**, 194.

Grossman, S.P. and Mountford, H. (1964) *Amer. J. Physiol.*, **207**, 1387.

Grossman, S.P. and Peters, R.H. (1966) *J. comp. physiol. Psych.*, **61**, 325.

Grossman, S.P., Peters, R.H., Freedman, P.E. and Willer, H.I. (1965) *J. comp. physiol. Psych.*, **59**, 57.

Guerrero-Figueroa, R. and Heath, R.G. (1964) *Arch. Neurol.*, **10**, 74.

Gunne, L.M. and Reis, D.J. (1963) *Life Sci.*, **11**, 804.

Hall, C.D., Buchwald, N.A. and Ling, G. (1968) *Brain Res.*, **6**, 22.

Harvey, J.A. and Lints, C.E. (1965) *Science*, **148**, 250.

Hayward, J.N. and Smith, W.K. (1963) *Arch. Neurol.*, **9**, 171.

Hayward, J.N., Fairchild, M.D. and Stuart, D.G. (1966) *Exp. Brain Res.*, **1**, 205.

Hilton, S.M. and Zbrozyna, A.W. (1963) *J. Physiol.*, 165, 160.
Horvath, F.E. (1963) *J. comp. physiol. Psych.*, 56, 380.
Hutchinson, R.R. and Renfrew, J.W. (1967) *J. comp. physiol. Psych.*, 63, 408.
Ibayashi, H., Uchikawa, T., Motohashi, K., Fujika, T., Yoshida, S., Ohsawa, N., Murakawa, S., Nakamara, N. and Okinaka, S. (1963) *Endocrinology*, 73, 816.
Ikeda, T. (1961) *Folia Psychiat. et Neurol. Jap.*, 15, 157.
Isaacson, R.L. and Wickelgren, W.O. (1962) *Science*, 138, 1104.
Jasper, H.H. and Koyama, I. (1968) *EEG clin. Neurophysiol.*, 24, 281.
Jasper, H.H., Ricci, G.F. and Doane, B. (1958) 'Patterns of cortical neuronal discharge during conditioned responses in monkeys' in *The Neurological Basis of Behaviour*. Ciba Foundation Symposium (G. E. W. Wolstenholme and C. M. O'Connor, eds.), London, Churchill.
Jefferson, Sir Geoffrey (1958) 'The reticular formation and clinical neurology' in *The Reticular Formation of the Brain* (H. H. Jasper and L. D. Proctor, eds.), London, Churchill.
John, E.R. (1961) *Ann. Rev. Physiol.*, 23, 451.
John, E.R. and Killam, K.F. (1959) *J. Pharm. exp. Therap.*, 125, 252.
John, E.R. and Killam, K.F. (1960) *J. nerv. ment. Dis.*, 131, 183.
Johnston, J.B. (1923) *J. comp. Neurol.*, 35, 337.
Kaada, B.R., Rasmussen, E.W. and Kveim, O. (1961) *Exp. Neurol.*, 3, 333.
Kaada, B.R., Rasmussen, E.W. and Kveim, O. (1962) *J. comp. physiol. Psych.*, 55, 661.
Kalynzhugi, L.V. (1964) *Fed. Proc. Trans. Supp.*, 23, 1733.
Kambach, M. (1967) *J. comp. physiol. Psych.*, 63, 231.
Kamikawa, K., McIlwain, J.T. and Adey, W.R. (1964) *EEG clin. Neurophysiol.*, 17, 485.
Kaplan, J. (1968) *J. comp. physiol. Psych.*, 65, 274.
Karmos, G. and Grastyán, E. (1962) *Acta Physiol. Acad. Sci. Hung.*, 21, 215.
Kavanar, J.L. (1964) *Science*, 143, 490.
Kawakami, M., Seto, K., Tevasawa, E. and Yoshida, K. (1967) *Prog. Brain Res.*, 27, 69.
Kawamura, H., Whitmoyer, D.I. and Sawyer, C.H. (1967) *EEG clin. Neurophysiol.*, 22, 337.
Key, B.J. (1965) *Nature*, 207, 441.
Killam, K.F. and Killam, E.K. (1967) *Prog. Brain Res.*, 27, 387.
Kimble, D.P. and Gostnell, D. (1968) *J. comp. physiol. Psych.*, 65, 290.
Kimble, D.P. and Kimble, R.J. (1965) *J. comp. physiol. Psych.*, 60, 474.
Kimble, D.P., Kirkby, R.J. and Stein, D.G. (1966) *J. comp. physiol. Psych.*, 61, 141.
Kimble, D.P. and Pribram, K.H. (1963) *Science*, 139, 824.
Kimble, D.P. and Rogers, L. (1967) *J. comp. physiol. Psych.*, 63, 401.

King, F.A. (1958) *J. nerv. ment. Dis.*, **126**, 57.

Kleist, K. (1934) 'Gehirn-Pathologie vornehurlich auf grund der Kreiges-fahrungen' in *Handbuch der ärzlichen Erfahrungen in Weltkreig*, Vol. 4, Leipzig, Barth.

Kling, A. (1962) *Science*, **137**, 429.

Kling, A. (1966) *Psychosomatic Med.*, **28**, 155.

Kling, A., Orbach, J., Schwartz, N.B. and Towne, J.C. (1960) *Arch. gen. Psychiat.*, **3**, 391.

Klüver, H. and Bucy, P.C. (1937) *Amer. J. Physiol.*, **119**, 352.

Klüver, H. and Bucy, P.C. (1938) *J. Psychol.*, **5**, 33.

Klüver, H. and Bucy, P.C. (1939) *Arch. Neurol. Psychiat.*, **42**, 979.

Knigge, K.M. (1961) *Proc. Soc. Exp. Biol. Med.*, **108**, 18.

Knigge, K.M. and Hays, M. (1963) *Proc. Soc. Exp. Biol. Med.*, **114**, 67.

Knott, J.R., Ingram, W.R. and Correll, R.E. (1960) *Arch. Neurol.*, **2**, 247 and 476.

Koikegami, H., Fuse, S., Hiroki, S., Kazami, T. and Kogeyama, Y. (1958) *Folia Psychiat. et Neurol. Jap.*, **12**, 207.

Kopa, J., Szabo, I. and Grastyán, E. (1962) *Acta Physiol. Acad. Sci. Hung.*, **21**, 207.

Laursen, A.M. (1962) *Dan. Med. Bull.*, **9**, 21.

Lesse, H. (1960) 'Rhinencephalic electrophysiological activity during "emotional behavior" in cats' in *Explorations in the Physiology of Emotions* (L. Jolyon West and M. Greenblatt, eds.). *A.P.A. Psychiat. Res. Reports*, **12**, 224.

Lesse, H., Heath, R.G., Mickle, W.A., Monroe, R.R. and Miller, W.H. (1955) *J. nerv. ment. Dis.*, **122**, 433.

Levison, P.K. and Flynn, J.P. (1965) *Animal Behaviour*, **13**, 217.

Lewis, P.R. and Shute, C.C.D. (1967) *Brain*, **90**, 521.

Lindsley, D.F., Carpenter, R.S., Killam, E.K. and Killam, K.F. (1968) *EEG clin. Neurophysiol.*, **24**, 497.

Lippold, O.C.J. and Redfearn, J.W.T. (1964) *Brit. J. Psychiat.*, **110**, 768.

Lissák, H. and Endröczi, E. (1961) 'Neurohumoral factors in the control of animal behaviour' in *Brain Mechanisms and Learning* (J. F. Delafresnaye, ed.), Oxford, Blackwell Scientific Publications.

Lissák, H. and Grastyán, E. (1957) *Proc. 1st. Intern. Congr. Neurol. Sci.*, Brussels.

Lorente de Nò, R. (1934) *J. Psychol. Neurol. (Leipzig)*, **46**, 113.

Lyon, M. (1964) *J. comp. Neurol.*, **122**, 407.

MacDonnell, M.F. and Flynn, J.P. (1966) *Science*, **152**, 1406.

MacKay, D.M. (1966) in *Brain and Conscious Experience* (J. C. Eccles, ed.), Berlin, Springer.

MacLean, P.D. (1955) *Psychosom. Med.*, **17**, 355.

McLennan, H. and Greystone, P. (1965) *Canad. J. Physiol. Pharm.*, **43**, 1009.

Manzoni, T. and Parmeggiani, P.L. (1964) *Helv. Physiol. Pharm. Acta*, **22**, C28.

Manzoni, T. and Parmeggiani, P.L. (1965) *Helv. Physiol. Pharm. Acta*, **23**, 180.

Mason, J.W., Nauta, W.J.H., Brady, J.V., Robinson, J.A., and Sachar, E.J. (1961) *Acta Neurovegitativa*, **23**, 4.

Meissner, W.W. (1968) *Int. J. Neuropsychiat.*, **4**, 6.

Miller, N.E., DiCara, L.V. and Wolf, G. (1968) *Amer. J. Physiol.*, **215**, 684.

Mirsky, A., Miller, R. and Steen, M. (1953) *Psychosom. Med.*, **15**, 574.

Misanin, J.R., Miller, R.R. and Lewis, D.J. (1968) *Science*, **160**, 554.

Moore, R.Y. (1964) *J. comp. physiol. Psychol.*, **57**, 65.

Moore, R.Y., Heller, A., Wurtman, R.J. and Axelrod, J. (1967) *Science*, **148**, 250.

Morrell, F. (1961) *Physiol. Rev.*, **41**, 443.

Murphy, J.T., Dreifuss, J.J. and Gloor, P. (1967) *Amer. J. Physiol.*, **214**, 1443.

Murphy, J.T., Dreifuss, J.J. and Gloor, P. (1968) *Brain Res.*, **8**, 167.

Myers, R.D. (1964) *Canad. J. Psychol.*, **18**, 6.

Nathan, P.W. and Smith, M.C. (1950) *J. Neurol. Neurosurg.*, *Psychiat.*, **13**, 191.

Narabayashi, H., Nagoa, T., Saito, Y., Yoshida, M. and Nagahata, M. (1963) *Arch. Neurol.*, **9**, 1.

Nauta, W.H. (1958) *Brain*, **81**, 319.

Nielson, H.C. and Fleming, R.M. (1968) *Exp. Neurol.*, **20**, 21.

Nielson, H.C., Knight, J.M. and Porter, P.B. (1962) *J. comp. physiol. Psychol.*, **55**, 168.

Nielson, H.C , McIver, A.H. and Boswell, R.S. (1965) *Exp. Neurol.*, **11**, 147.

Olds, J. (1958) 'Adaptive functions of paleocortical and related structures' in *The Biological and Biochemical Basis of Behavior* (H. F. Harlow and C. N. Woolsey, eds.), Madison, University of Wisconsin Press.

Olds, J. (1959) *Ann. Rev. Physiol.*, **21**, 381.

Olds, J. and Olds, M.E. (1961) 'Interference and learning in paleocortical systems' in *Brain Mechanisms and Learning* (J. F. Delafresnaye, ed.), Oxford, Blackwell Scientific Publications.

Olds, M.E. and Olds, J. (1963) *J. Comp. Neurol.*, **120**, 259.

Olds, J., Yuwiler, A., Olds, M.E. and Yun, C. (1964) *Amer. J. Physiol.*, **207**, 242.

Olton, D.S. and Isaacson, R.L. (1967) *J. comp. physiol. Psychol.*, **64**, 256.

Orbach, J., Milner, B. and Rasmussen, T. (1960) *Arch. Neurol.*, **3**, 230.

O'Steen, W.K. and Vaughan, G.M. (1968) *Brain Res.*, **8**, 209.

Pagni, C.A. and Marossero, F. (1965) *EEG clin. Neurophysiol.*, **18**, 260.

Papez, J.W. (1937) *Arch. Neurol. Psychiat.*, **38**, 725.

Parmeggiani, P.L. and Rabini, C. (1964) *Helv. Physiol. Pharm. Acta*, **22**, C31.

Pechtel, C., McAvoy, T., Levitt, M., Kling, A. and Masserman, J.H. (1958) *J. nerv. ment. Dis.*, **126**, 148.

Peretz, E. (1960) *J. comp. physiol. Psychol.*, **53**, 540.

Petsche, H. and Stumpf, C. (1960) *EEG clin. Neurophysiol.*, **12**, 589.

Petsche, H., Stumpf, C. and Gogolak, G. (1962) *EEG clin. Neurophysiol.*, **14**, 202.

Phillis, J.W. (1968) *Brain Res.*, **7**, 378.

Phillis, J.W. and York, D.H. (1967) *Brain Res.*, **5**, 517.

Pickenhain, L. and Klingberg, F. (1967) *Prog. Brain Res.*, **27**, 218.

Plante, S. (1969) Personal Communication.

Pool, J.L. (1954) *J. Neurosurg.*, **11**, 45.

Porter, R., Adey, W.R. and Brown, T.S. (1964) *Exp. Neurol.*, **10**, 216.

Poschel, B.P.H. and Ninteman, F.W. (1963) *Life Sci.*, **10**, 782.

Poschel, B.P.H. and Ninteman, F.W. (1968) *Life Sci.*, **7**, 317.

Pribram, K.H. and Weiskrantz, L. (1955) paper read to the Eastern Psychological Association, April, 1955: quoted by Olds, J. (1958) in *The Biological and Biochemical Basis of Behavior* (H. F. Harlow and C. N. Woolsey, eds.), Madison, University of Wisconsin Press, p. 261.

Rabe, A. and Haddad, R.K. (1968) *Exp. Brain Res.*, **5**, 259.

Radulovacki, M. and Adey, W.R. (1965) *Exp. Neurol.*, **12**, 68.

Raisman, G. (1966) *Brit. Med. Bull.*, **22**, 197.

Reis, D.J. and Fuxe, K. (1968) *Brain Res.*, **7**, 448.

Riss, W., Burstein, S.D. and Johnston, R.W. (1963) *Amer. J. Physiol.*, **203**, 861.

Richardson, A.J. and Glow, P.H. (1967) *J. comp. physiol. Psychol.*, **63**, 240.

Roberts, W.W. and Carey, R.J. (1963) *J. comp. physiol. Psychol.*, **56**, 950.

Roberts, W.W., Denber, W.N. and Brodwick, M. (1962) *J. comp. physiol. Psychol.*, **55**, 695.

Robinson, E. (1963) *J. comp. physiol. Psychol.*, **56**, 814.

Rodgers, W.L., Epstein, A.N. and Teitelbaum, P. (1965) *Amer. J. Physiol.*, **208**, 334.

Rosenzweig, M.R. (1966) *American Psychologist*, **21**, 321.

Rosvold, H.E., Mirsky, A.F. and Pribram, K.H. (1954) *J. comp. physiol. Psychol.*, **47**, 173.

Rosvold, H.E. and Mishkin, M. (1961) 'Non-sensory effects of frontal lesions on discrimination learning and performance' in *Brain Mechanisms and Learning* (J. F. Delafresnaye, ed.), Oxford, Blackwell Scientific Publications.

Rubin, B.M. (1968) *EEG clin. Neurophysiol.*, **25**, 344.

Rubin, B.M. (1968) *EEG clin. Neurophysiol.*, **25**, 344.

Rubin, R.J., Mandell, A.J. and Crandall, P.H. (1966) *Science*, **153**, 767.

Schachter, S. and Singer, J.E. (1962) *Psychol. Rev.*, **69**, 379.

Schiff, B.B. (1967) *J. comp. physiol. Psychol.*, **64**, 16.

Schreiner, L. and Kling, A. (1954) *Arch. Neurol. Psychiat.*, **72**, 180.

Schwartzbaum, J.S. (1960) *J. comp. physiol. Psychol.*, **53**, 388.

Schwartzbaum, J.S. (1965) *J. comp. physiol. Psychol.*, **60**, 314.

Schwartzbaum, J.S. and Gay, P.E. (1966) *J. comp. physiol. Psychol.*, **61**, 59.

Schwartzbaum, J.S., Green, R.H., Beatty, W.W. and Thompson, J.B. (1967) *J. comp. physiol. Psychol.*, **63**, 95.

Schwartzbaum, J.S., Kellicuff, M.H., Spieth, T.M. and Thompson, J.B. (1964a) *J. comp. physiol. Psychol.*, **58**, 217.

Schwartzbaum, J.S., Thompson, J.B. and Kellicuff, M.H. (1964b) *J. comp. physiol. Psychol.*, **57**, 257.

Scoville, W.B. (1954) *J. Neurosurg.*, **11**, 64.

Sem-Jacobsen, C.W. and Torkildsen, A. (1960) 'Depth recording and electrical stimulation in the human brain' in *Electrical Studies on the Unanesthetized Brain* (E. R. Ramsey and D. S. O'Doherty, eds.), New York, Hoeber.

Sheard, M.H. and Aghajanian, G.K. (1968) *Life Sci.*, **7**, 19.

Shute, C.C.D. and Lewis, P.R. (1967) *Brain*, **90**, 497.

Siegal, A. and Flynn, J.P. (1968) *Brain Res.*, **7**, 252.

Singer, G. and Montgomery, R.B. (1968) *Science*, **160**, 1017.

Singh, D., Johnston, H.J. and Klosterman, H.J. (1967) *Nature*, **216**, 1337.

Slotnick, B.M. (1967) *Behaviour*, **29**, 204.

Soulairac, A., Gottesman, G. and Charpentier, J. (1967) *Int. J. Neuropharm.*, **6**, 71.

Spiegel, E.A., Miller, H.R. and Oppenheimer, M.J. (1940) *J. Neurophysiol.*, **3**, 538.

Sprague, J.M., Levitt, M., Robson, K., Liu, C.N., Stellar, E. and Chambers, W.W. (1963) *Arch. Ital. Biol.*, **101**, 225.

Stein, D.G. and Kimble, D.P. (1966) *J. comp. physiol. Psychol.*, **62**, 243.

Stepien, L.S., Cordeau, J.P. and Rasmussen, T. (1960) *Brain*, **83**, 470.

Stevens, D.A., Resnick, O. and Krus, D.M. (1967) *Life Sci.*, **6**, 2215.

Stumpf, C. (1965) *Int. Rev. Neurobiol.*, **8**, 77.

Swanson, A.M. and Isaacson, R.L. (1967) *J. comp. physiol. Psychol.*, **64**, 30.

Teitelbaum, H. and Milner, P. (1963) *J. comp. physiol. Psychol.*, **56**, 284.

Terzian, H. and Ore, G.D. (1955) *Neurology*, **5**, 373.

Thiery, A.M., Javoy, F., Glowinski, J. and Kety, S.S. (1968) *J. Neurochem.*, **15**, 163.

Thomas, G.J., Fry, W.J., Fry, F.J., Slotnick, B.M. and Krickhaus, E.E. (1963) *J. Neurophysiol.*, **26**, 857.

Thomas, G.J., Moore, R.Y., Harvey, J.A. and Hunt, H.F. (1959) *J. comp. physiol. Psychol.*, **52**, 527.

Thomas, G.J. and Otis, L.S. (1958a) *J. comp. physiol. Psychol.*, **51**, 130.

Thomas, G.J. and Otis, L.S. (1958b) *J. comp. physiol. Psychol.*, **51**, 161.

Thomas, G.J. and Slotnick, B.M. (1962) *J. comp. physiol. Psychol.*, **55**, 1085.

Thomas, G.J. and Slotnick, B.M. (1963) *J. comp. physiol. Psychol.*, **56**, 959.

Thompson, R. (1963) *J. comp. physiol. Psychol.*, **56**, 261.

Thompson, R., Langer, S.K. and Rich, I. (1964) *Brain*, **87**, 537.

Thompson, R. and Hawkins, W.F. (1961) *Exp. Neurol.*, **3**, 189.

Thompson, R. and Rich, I. (1961) *Exp. Neurol.*, **4**, 310.

Travis, R.P. Jr., Sparks, D.L. and Hooten, T.F. (1968) *Brain Res.*, **7**, 455.

Ursin, H. (1965) *Exp. Neurol.*, **11**, 298.

References 179

Ursin, H. and Kaada, B.R. (1960a) *Exp. Neurol.*, **2**, 109.

Ursin, H. and Kaada, B.R. (1960b) *EEG clin. Neurophysiol.*, **12**, 1.

Valenstein, E.S. (1968) *Neurosciences Res. Prog. Bull.*, **6**, 85.

Valenstein, E.S., Cox, V.C. and Kakolewski, J.W. (1968) *Science*, **159**, 1119.

Valenstein, E.S. and Valenstein, T. (1964) *Science*, **145**, 1456.

Vanderwolf, C.H. and Heron, W. (1964) *Arch. Neurol.*, **11**, 379.

Victor, M., Angevine, J.B., Mancall, E.L. and Fisher, C.M. (1961) *Arch. Neurol.*, **5**, 244.

Votaw, C.L. (1960) *J. comp. Neurol.*, **114**, 283.

Walter, W. Grey (1965) Personal Communication.

Walter, W. Grey, Cooper, R., Aldridge, V.J., McCallum, W.C. and Winter, A.L. (1964) *Nature*, **203**, 280.

Webster, D.B. and Voneida, T.J. (1964) *Exp. Neurol.*, **10**, 170.

Weiskrantz, L. (1956) *J. comp. physiol. Psychol.*, **4**, 381.

Weiskrantz, L. (1958) quoted by H. D. Patton, *Amer. Rev. Physiol.*, **20**, 509.

Wepsic, J.G. and Sutin, J. (1964) *Exp. Neurol.*, **10**, 67.

Wheatley, M.D. (1944) *Arch. Neurol. Psychiat.*, **52**, 296.

Wickelgren, W.O. and Isaacson, R.L. (1963) *Nature*, **200**, 48.

Winocur, G. and Salzen, E.A. (1968) *J. comp. physiol. Psychol.*, **65**, 303.

Wood, C.D. (1958) *Neurology*, **8**, 215.

Wurtz, R.H. (1965) *EEG clin. Neurophysiol.*, **18**, 649 and **19**, 521.

Wurtz, R.H. (1966) *EEG clin. Neurophysiol.*, **20**, 59.

Wurtz, R.H. and Olds, J. (1963) *J. comp. physiol. Psychol.*, **56**, 941.

Yamaguchi, Y., Yoshii, N., Miyamoto, K. and Itoigawa, N. (1967) *Prog. Brain Res.*, **27**, 281.

Yamamoto, C. and Kawai, N. (1967) *Exp. Neurol.*, **19**, 176.

Yasukochi, G., Haruta, Y. and Tsutsuimi, S. (1962) *Folia Psychiat. et Neurol. Jap.*, **16**, 159.

Yokata, T. and Fujimori, B. (1964) *EEG clin. Neurophysiol.* **16**, 375.

Zeman, W. and King, F.A. (1958) *J. nerv. ment. Dis.*, **127**, 490.

AUTHOR INDEX

Adey W.R. 6, 8, 10, 18, 29, 44, 92,
    95, 102, 103, 104, 105, 108,
    109, 110, 116, 121, 126, 127,
    147, 170, 172, 174, 177
Aghajanian G.K. 141, 178
Akert K. 44, 170
Allen W.F. 63, 170
Allikinets L.H. 53, 61, 170
Altman J. 133, 170
Anand B.K. 81, 170
Anderson P. 28, 170
Andersson B. 170
Aprison M.H. 141, 170
Arbit J. 70, 172

Bagshaw M.H. 50, 58, 170
Baile C.A. 140, 170
Baird N.H. 90, 170
Baker W.W. 138, 170
Barbizet J. 75, 170
Bard P. 46, 47, 170
Barker D.J. 100, 170
Barondes S.H. 131, 170
Bar-Sela M.E. 52, 170
Benedict F. 138, 170
Benzies S. 50, 170
Biscoe T.J. 139, 170
Bizzi E. 81, 170
Bleier R. 35, 170
Boehlke K.W. 137, 172
Bohus B. 59, 89, 170, 172
Bond D.D. 79, 170
Brady J.V. 64, 76, 91, 144, 170, 171,
    176
Brazier M.A.B. 71, 150, 171
Bremner F.J. 106, 171
Brobeck J.R. 81, 170
Bromiley R.B. 81, 171
Brown B.B. 105, 171
Brown S. 44, 171

Brutowski S. 54, 171
Buchwald N.A. 9, 51, 171, 173
Bucy P.C. 5, 43, 62, 63, 175
Bunnell B.N. 78, 171
Bureš J. 87, 171
Burešová O. 30, 63, 87, 171
Burkett E.E. 78, 171

Carey R.J. 90, 91, 171, 177
Chance M. 47, 171
Chapman W.R. 62, 171
Chase M.H. 108, 171
Chatrian G.E. 62, 171
Chow K.L. 96, 171
Clark C.V.H. 68, 171
Cohen H.D. 131, 170
Conrad D.G. 91, 171
Coons E.E. 81, 171
Coppock H.W. 58, 170
Correll R.E. 67, 70, 171, 175
Critchelow V. 52, 170

Dahl D 83, 171
Delgado J.M.R. 55, 80, 143, 144,
    153, 156, 171
Deutsch J.A. 126, 132, 171
de Wied D. 89, 170, 171
Diamond M.C. 134, 171
Dicara L.V. 82, 172, 176
Domino E.F. 137, 138, 172
Donovan B.T. 81, 172
Douglas R.J. 64, 78, 172
Drachman D.A. 69, 70, 172
Dreifuss J.J. 35, 52, 172

Egger M.D. 50, 80, 172
Ehrlich A. 82, 172
Elazar Z. 105, 172

Eleftheriou E. 137, 172
Ellen P. 71, 72, 77, 79, 172
Elliott Smith G. 14, 15, 172
Elul R. 31, 172
Endröczi E. 57, 58, 60, 71, 77, 84, 172, 175
Ervin F.R. 9, 51, 171

Feldberg W. 141, 172
Feldman S. 85, 111, 172
Fendler K. 59, 172
Fernandez de Molina A. 51, 55, 172
Fleming R.M. 137, 176
Flynn J.P. 50, 71, 80, 85, 172, 175, 178
Folkow B. 81, 172
Fonberg E. 56, 171, 172
Fraschini F. 140, 172
Freeman W.J. 126, 172
Fujimori B. 107, 179
Fuller J.L. 46, 172
Fuxe K. 81, 136, 172, 177

Galambos R. 10, 172
Gastaut H. 5, 83, 86, 172
Gay P.E. 78, 79, 177
Gergen J.A. 28, 173
Gloor P. 28, 52, 143, 173
Glow P.H. 132, 177
Goddard G.V. 58, 173
Gostnell D. 100, 174
Grant L.D. 29, 74, 173
Grastyán E. 64, 106, 107, 109, 116, 123, 151, 173, 174, 175
Green J.D. 5, 29, 45, 46, 47, 63, 70, 109, 173, 177
Gregory R. 9, 173
Greystone P. 110, 175
Grossman S.P. 51, 69, 79, 88, 89, 173
Guerrero-Figueroa R. 108, 173
Gunne L.M. 60, 173

Haddad R.K. 68, 177
Hall C.D. 140, 173
Harvey J.A. 142, 173

Hawkins W.F. 84, 178
Hays M. 76, 175
Hayward J.N. 59, 121, 173
Heath R.G. 108, 175
Heron W. 105, 179
Hilton S.M. 51, 174
Himwich H.E. 4, 16, 24, 148
Hingtgen J.N. 141, 170
Horvath F.E. 53, 54, 174
Hunsperger R.W. 51, 55, 172
Hutchinson R.R. 140, 174

Ibayashi H. 59, 174
Ikeda T. 53, 174
Isaacson R.L. 63, 67, 68, 90, 171, 174, 176, 179

Jarrard L.E. 29, 74, 173
Jasper H.H. 127, 139, 174
Jefferson, Sir Geoffrey 79, 174
John E.R. 110, 111, 124, 146, 174

Kaada B.R. 50, 63, 76, 84, 174, 179
Kalynzhugi L.V. 137, 174
Kambach M. 69, 174
Kamikawa K. 83, 174
Kaplan J. 69, 174
Karmos G. 64, 172, 173, 174
Kavanar J.L. 89, 174
Kawai N. 138, 179
Kawakami M. 59, 174
Kawamura H. 120, 174
Key B.J. 114, 174
Killam E.K. 61, 174, 175
Killam K.F. 61, 110, 111, 123, 174, 175
Kimble D.P. 68, 72, 74, 100, 174
Kimble R.J. 68, 174
King F.A. 53, 76, 77, 79, 175, 179
Kleist K. 143, 175
Kling A. 45, 46, 47, 53, 59, 175, 177
Klingberg F. 103, 177
Klüver H. 5, 43, 62, 63, 175
Knigge K.M. 57, 75, 175
Knott J.R. 71, 83, 88, 90, 171, 175

Koikegami H. 59, 175
Kopa J. 88, 175
Koyama I. 139, 174

Lapin I.P. 53, 61, 170
Laursen A.M. 91, 175
Lesse H. 8, 108, 109, 147, 175
Lewis P.R. 138, 139, 175, 177
Lindsley D.F. 92, 124, 175
Lints C.E. 142, 173
Lippold O.C.J. 120, 175
Lissák H. 57, 58, 60, 71, 77, 84, 123, 172, 175
Lorente de Nò R. 29, 175
Lutsky H. 132, 171
Lyon M. 87, 175

MacDonnell M.F. 85, 175
MacKay D.M. 156, 175
MacLean P.D. 4, 24, 28, 87, 173, 175
McLennan H. 110, 175
Manzoni T. 108, 175, 176
Marossero F. 109, 176
Mason J.W. 57, 176
Meissner W.W. 134, 176
Miller N.E. 132, 171, 176
Mirsky A., 60, 176, 177
Misanin J.R. 130, 176
Mishkin 8, 177
Montgomery R.B. 140, 178
Moore R.Y. 63, 77, 142, 176, 178
Morrel F. 10, 118, 126, 176
Mountcastle V.B. 46, 47, 170
Murphy J.T. 35, 52, 83, 172, 176
Myers R.D. 141, 176

Narabayashi H. 62, 176
Nathan P.W. 151, 176
Nauta W.H. 8, 176
Nielson H.C. 78, 79, 130, 131, 137, 176
Ninteman F.W. 137, 142, 177

Olds J. 84, 87, 137, 144, 154, 176, 179
Olds M.E. 84, 87, 137, 172, 176
Olton D.S. 90, 176
Orbach J. 47, 176
Ommaya A.K. 69, 172
Ore G.D. 48, 178
O'Steen W.K. 142, 176
Otis L.S. 63, 99, 100, 178

Pagni C.A. 109, 176
Papez J.W. 5, 6, 29, 33, 143, 176
Parmeggiani P.L. 108, 119, 175, 176
Pechtel C. 98, 176
Peretz E. 99, 176
Peters R.H. 88, 173
Petsche H. 76, 105, 176, 177
Phillis J.W. 138, 139, 177
Pickenhain L. 103, 177
Plante S. 40, 177
Pool J.L. 63, 177
Porter R. 104, 177
Poschel P.B.H. 137, 142, 177
Powell E.W. 71, 72, 79, 172
Pribram K.H. 53, 63, 72, 172, 174, 177

Rabe A. 68, 177
Rabini C. 119, 176
Radulovacki M. 108, 177
Raisman G. 32, 171, 177
Raphelson A.C. 78, 172
Redfearn J.W.T. 120, 175
Reis D.J. 60, 81, 173, 177
Renfrew J.W. 140, 174
Rich I. 40, 178
Richardson A.J. 132, 177
Riss W. 59, 177
Roberts W.W. 90, 177
Robinson E. 53, 177
Rocklin K.W. 132, 171
Rodgers W.L. 81, 177
Rosenzweig M.R. 134, 171, 177
Rosvold H.E. 8, 10, 46, 172, 177
Rubin B.M. 82, 177

Rubin R.J. 57, 177
Rubinstein E.H. 81, 172
Salzen E.A. 67, 179
Schachter S. 138, 177
Schaeffer E.A. 44, 171
Schiff B.V. 87, 177
Schreiner L. 45, 47, 177
Schwartzbaum J.S. 54, 55, 78, 79, 177, 178
Scoville W.B. 63, 67, 171, 178
Sem-Jacobsen C.W. 95, 178
Sheard M.H. 141, 178
Shute C.C.D. 138, 139, 178
Siegal A. 71, 178
Silverman P. 47, 171
Singer G. 140, 178
Singer J.E. 138, 177
Singh D. 134, 178
Slotnick B.M. 99, 100, 178
Smith W.K. 59, 151, 173
Soulairac A. 74, 178
Spiegel E.A. 47, 76, 178
Sprague J.M. 87, 178
Stein D.G. 68, 178
Stepien L.S. 45, 63, 178
Stevens D.A. 142, 178
Straughan D.W. 139, 170
Stumpf C. 105, 139, 176, 178
Sutin J. 110, 179
Swanson A.M. 68, 178

Terzian H. 48, 178
Thiery A.M. 138, 178
Thomas G.J. 63, 77, 99, 100, 178
Thompson R. 40, 69, 84, 88, 90, 178

Torkildsen A. 95, 178
Travis R.P. 91, 178

Ursin H. 50, 54, 178, 179

Valenstein E.S. 81, 89, 179
Valenstein T. 89, 179
Vanderwolf C.H. 105, 179
Vaughan G.M. 142, 176
Victor M. 74, 179
Votaw C.L. 29, 179

Walter W. Grey 115, 120, 121, 160, 179
Webster D.B. 68, 72, 164, 179
Weiskrantz L. 11, 47, 53, 54, 63, 177, 179
Wepsic J.G. 110, 179
Wheatley M.D. 80, 179
Wickelgren W.O. 63, 67, 174, 179
Winocur G. 67, 179
Wolf G. 82, 172, 176, 179
Wood C.D. 46, 179
Wurtz R.H. 121, 154, 179

Yamaguchi Y. 108, 179
Yamamoto C. 138, 179
Yasukochi G. 63, 179
Yokata T. 107, 179
York D.H. 138, 177

Zbrozyna A.W. 51, 174
Zeman W. 79, 179

SUBJECT INDEX

ACTH 57–60, 84, 133
Aggressive behaviour 46–48, 49, 50–53, 60–62, 71, 76, 79, 80–82, 87, 98–99, 137, 140, 152–153
Alzheimer's disease 75
Amygdala
anatomy 20
connections 29, 31–34
function of 48–63, 76, 152–157
in human studies 61–63
fast rhythm 109–110
Antidiuretic hormone 59, 132–133
Arousal 74, 86, 113–114, 138, 151

Basal ganglia 90–92
Bechterew's nucleus 38

Cholinergic neurones 36, 74, 88, 109, 126, 132, 137, 138–140
Cingulate cortex 41, 59–60, 66, 96–101
Cingulum 28, 41
Conditioned emotional response 66, 99
Conditioned reflexes 53, 63–66, 77, 79, 83–85, 86–90, 91–92, 99–101, 113f, 122–123, 152, 153–154
stages of formation 113–123
Contingent negative variation 120, 150, 160

Delusions, origins of 159–166
Depression 158–160
Dominant locus 119–121
Dopamine neurons 36, 137
Drinking behaviour 51, 53, 79, 89, 121, 140–141

ECT
effects on memory 129–131
Entorhinal area 29, 93
Epilepsy 119
Epilepsy, temporal lobe 62, 70, 87, 93–95, 112
Ethology 47

Feeding behaviour 51, 53, 56, 58, 79, 81–82, 89, 91, 121, 128, 140–141
Feldman's hypothesis 85, 86, 111–112
Fornix 23, 25–28, 34, 75, 102, 151
Freud 162–163, 167–168
Frontal cortex 150

Glutamate 139–140
Gudden's nuclei 38

Habenula 35, 41
Hippocampus
anatomy 16–20
connections 25–31, 76
wiring diagram 27–28, 147–148
theta rhythm 29, 76, 86, 102–109, 115–117, 139
function of 63–75, 104–109, 114, 138, 144, 145–152
congenital absence 151–152
Hypothalamus 29, 30
connections 34–36, 83
functions of 80–86, 140–141, 152
Hypersexuality 45, 47, 52, 57, 84

Imipramine 61
Impedance 121–122
Interpeduncular nucleus 40

Intralaminar thalamic nuclei 40–41, 115, 119
function of 88–89
Iron, ions as cause of artefacts 82
Isohippocampal rhythm 108

Klüver-Bucy syndrome 5, 43–48
in humans 48, 63
Konorski's compound stimulus test 63–64, 66–67
Korsakoff, syndrome 63, 75, 134–135

Learning
electrical concomitants 102–109, 110, 114, 118–121, 147
role of amygdala 53–57, 60f, 125–138, 153
role of basal ganglia 91
role of cingulate gyrus 99—101
role of hippocampus 63–75, 125–128
role of hypothalamus 83–85, 125–128
role of neocortex 123–124
role of reticular formation 86–87, 125–128
role of septum 77–79, 125–128
role of subthalamic area 92–93
role of thalamic nuclei 88–90
Limbic system
development 13–17
olfactory connections 25
Locus coerulus 136
LSD 61, 109, 139, 141

Maternal behaviour 74, 100–101
Medial forebrain bundle 25, 32, 35, 136, 137
Memory 44–45, 48, 65f, 79, 86–87, 94–95, 98, 108, 119, 145f, 155
mechanism 129–135
role of acetylcholine 132–133
role of protein synthesis 131
Motivation 69–89, 107, 144

Neurosciences Research Program 3
Neurosis
physiological basis 163–169
Norepinephrine neurons 36, 60–61, 74, 80, 136–138, 160

Orbitofrontal cortex 41, 96–101
Orienting reflex 64–65, 106, 114–116, 117
Ovarian function 58–59

Papez circuit 5, 75, 146
PCPA 141
Pituitary 35, 57–60, 76, 88, 110, 133, 151, 155
Pyriform lobe 23, 31, 57

Raphe nuclei 136, 141–142
Reinforcement control of 55, 87
Respiration 96
Reticular formulation,
anatomy 36–40
function of 71, 86–87, 92, 102–105, 114f, 124–125, 139, 143, 144, 146f, 153
Reward centres 52, 56, 84, 89, 137, 154

Schaeffer collaterals 28
Schizophrenia 1, 2, 165–167
Searching response 50–88, 153
Septum 102,
anatomy 208–23, 2
connections 33–34, 76
function of 75–80, 138, 144
Sleep 91, 93, 108, 137, 138, 141
Serotonin neurones 36, 136, 141–142, 160
'Split-brain' preparations 72–73
Steady potentials 118–121
Steroids 57, 76, 85
Stimulus discrimination 44, 54–55
Stress 137–138
Stria medullaris 23–24, 32, 34

Stria terminalis   24, 32, 35, 51
Subthalamus   28, 29, 92–93, 151

Temperature regulation   85
Temporal discrimination   71–72
Temporal neocortex   41, 93–96, 150

Thalamic nuclei
   dorsomedial nucleus   89–90
   anterior nuclei   90
Tsai's vental tegmental area   38

Zona incerta   72